Why Psychiatry Is
a Branch of Medicine

Why Psychiatry Is a Branch of Medicine

SAMUEL B. GUZE, M.D.
Spencer T. Olin Professor of Psychiatry
Washington University School of Medicine
St. Louis, Missouri

New York   Oxford
OXFORD UNIVERSITY PRESS
1992

Oxford University Press

Oxford   New York   Toronto
Delhi   Bombay   Calcutta   Madras   Karachi
Kuala Lumpur   Singapore   Hong Kong   Tokyo
Nairobi   Dar es Salaam   Cape Town
Melbourne   Auckland

and associated companies in
Berlin   Ibadan

Copyright © 1992 by Oxford University Press, Inc.

Published by Oxford University Press, Inc.
200 Madison Avenue, New York, New York 10016

Library of Congress Cataloging-in-Publication Data
Guze, Samuel B. 1923–
Why psychiatry is a branch of medicine / Samuel B. Guze.
p.   cm.   Includes bibliographical references and index.
ISBN 0-19-507420-3
1. Psychiatry—Philosophy.   I. Title.
[DNLM: 1. Medicine.   2. Psychiatry.   WM 21 G993W]
RC437.5.G89   1992
616.89'001—dc20
DNLM/DLC
for Library of Congress   92-6001

1 3 5 7 9 8 6 4 2

Printed in the United States of America
on acid-free paper

To Charlotte, Chloe, Thea, Tessa, and Samantha:
My splendid connections to the future

PREFACE

Throughout many years in psychiatry, I have been thinking about and working to understand the relationship of psychiatric disorders to general medicine. In fact, I can remember several discussions with my teachers in internal medicine, Barry Wood and Carl Moore, in which I tried to explain the reasons for my decision to shift from internal medicine to psychiatry. Perhaps the main reason was to help incorporate into psychiatry some of the thinking associated with medicine generally, and with internal medicine specifically, in particular its emphasis on the central importance of diagnosis.

At the same time, I recognize that my ideas were shaped in many important ways by my colleagues in psychiatry, Eli Robins and George Winokur. All three of us were trying to clarify our thinking about psychiatric disorders and develop a viewpoint that would be convincing when taught and would lead to useful research.

I have pursued this goal with unflagging enthusiasm and commitment in my research and teaching. In papers and talks over the years, I've made continuous efforts to sharpen my thinking about psychiatric problems. Early on, I proposed that the best way of approaching psychiatric problems is to follow what I called *the medical model*. This will be characterized in detail in the following chapters.

Even though my views have evolved through the years, the basic concepts have remained the same. In this book, I've drawn together the various elements of my arguments and beliefs about psychiatry and tried to integrate them into a more comprehensive synthesis than was possible in earlier publications. I hope, of course, that this effort will be useful to other psychiatrists and the many students of psychiatry, both those who will become psychiatrists and those who will specialize in other areas of medicine.

I hope also that it may prove helpful to people outside medicine who are interested in the field and want to learn more about the medical approach to psychiatry. Today, medicine, including psychiatry, is of great interest to the public at large. Yet I have been impressed repeatedly by the difficulties even well-educated individuals experience in trying to understand the field. Trying to give these individuals a useful view of psychiatry is one of the goals of this book.

In addition, I hope the book will be read by philosophers, at least those interested in epistemology and in the mind-brain problem. It seems to me that psychiatric illness and the experiences of psychiatric patients raise important issues for philosophers of the mind and epistemologists. Just as philosophers have found it helpful, and perhaps even necessary, to try to deal with physics and evolution in their efforts to formulate and critique philosophical theories, so it may be helpful, and again perhaps necessary, for them to deal with psychiatric problems and observations.

This book is not long. I have tried throughout to concentrate on the most significant questions and concepts, but I don't pretend to have satisfactory answers for all these questions. My aim is not to present a guide to all of psychiatry. Instead, it has been to discuss the issues that seem of greatest importance at this point in the evolution of psychiatric thinking and practice. When we have learned more about psychiatric disorders, it will almost certainly be necessary to revise many of the discussions I have set forth. That is not at all disturbing to me—it will be a sign of professional progress.

New findings, new concepts, new approaches: they show that the field is developing and growing in wisdom. There is truly no room for complacency or dogmatism in psychiatry; it is much too important a subject for such attitudes to be accepted without a fight.

St. Louis   S.B.G.
January 1992

ACKNOWLEDGMENTS

"No man is an island" is the oft quoted admonition by John Donne. This is certainly true for any individual's efforts at setting down the ideas that have developed in his or her intellectual life. I know that my own ideas have been profoundly influenced over the years by an enormous number and range of people, living and dead. In fact, I believe that it is usually not possible to recognize fully one's intellectual debt. While this seems to be unavoidable, it is to be regretted.

I know that only some, perhaps only a very small part, of my ideas can be considered truly original; much of what I think and believe, including what follows in this book, is the result of absorbing, debating, and integrating the ideas and work of others. I have tried in this book and in my previous publications to cite people and work that have contributed to my current views. I may have left some out, but it was not intentional.

I also want to acknowledge with gratitude the incalculable debt I owe to my colleagues, students, and residents, who over the years through discussions, questions, arguments, and challenges forced me to try to clarify my thinking as much as possible. They have helped me more than I can ever truly acknowledge.

I must recognize especially my wife, Joy, whose confidence in me provided unflagging support for all that I have done. There is no way to measure properly the enormous generosity that has always characterized her approach to me and our marriage. I know of no way to thank her enough or appropriately.

I also want to express my gratitude to my institution, the Washington University School of Medicine. It educated me, trained me, and offered me the opportunity to be a member of its faculty and administration. It permitted and encouraged me to explore and cultivate my interests and talents without hindrance. It rewarded me in all the ways a medical school can. No medical school could have done more.

I must express my appreciation for the wonderful recommendations, suggestions, and support, over the many years we've worked together, from Jeff House, editor and friend, but especially for his excellent advice concerning the manuscript of this book.

Lastly, I want to thank my marvelous secretary, Rita Halpin, who has made my professional life so much easier for so many years. Cheerful, helpful, intelligent, and conscientious, she has been a tremendous asset throughout.

CONTENTS

Why Psychiatry Is
a Branch of Medicine

1

The Medical Model

Psychiatry is an intriguing field. It deals with the most characteristically human problems in all of medicine. It is concerned with disturbances in our sense of self, our relations with the rest of our world, our perceptions, our memories, our ability to think and judge, our motives and needs, our temperament and personality, our self evaluation, our sense of achievement and failure, our sexuality and capacity to respond to others and to love, our fears and moods, our compulsions and ruminations, our ability to communicate, and much more. What could be more exciting or more challenging!

At the same time, however, psychiatry can be frustrating and sometimes discouraging because it involves difficult and too often confusing concepts and methods. In addition, psychiatry can be demanding and even disappointing because our current capacities for truly effective intervention on behalf of our patients are still lacking in many ways and need much further advancement, even if they do represent significant progress from what was possible in the recent past. The primary motives for trying to understand more about psychiatric conditions are not simply to satisfy one's curiosity and receive greater intellectual stimulation, as important as these have been to many of us throughout our careers, but to be able to do a much better job with our patients. Many who share these views are committed to psychiatric research for the same reasons. Psychiatric disorders cause a tremendous amount of suffering to patients as well as to their families and friends. We need to do very much better, and clearer thinking and first-rate research are essential to accomplish this goal.

Psychiatry, more than any other branch of medicine, forces its practitioners to wrestle with the nature of evidence, the validity of introspec-

3

tion, problems in communication, and other long-standing philosophical issues. These issues make the field both frustrating and exciting.
Many scientists and physicians, including some psychiatrists, tend to
think somewhat disparagingly about philosophical matters as they touch
on science and medicine. This is unfortunate because philosophical
questions arise in all fields of science and medicine, and in psychiatry
they cannot be avoided. If we do not deal with them explicitly and
thoughtfully, psychiatric thinking and hence practice suffer.

Psychiatry is the branch of medicine devoted to the study and treatment of disorders in mental or psychological functions, which are also
referred to as psychopathology. Obviously, many disciplines, including
psychology, social work, theology, the law, philosophy, and others, are
also interested in these disorders. Each of these disciplines has a characteristic approach to psychopathology, but only psychiatry, as a medical specialty, offers the basis for a comprehensive approach from the
medical perspective. This medical perspective is what is meant when
we propose applying the medical model to psychiatric conditions. This
means simply that the concepts, strategies, and jargon of general medicine are applied to psychiatric disorders: diagnosis, differential diagnosis,
etiology, pathogenesis, treatment, natural history, epidemiology, complications, and so on.

Definition of Disease

Any discussion of the medical model and psychiatric disorders immediately raises questions about whether or not psychiatric conditions are
"real" diseases. The reason for this is obvious: if psychiatric conditions
are diseases, approaching them the way other diseases are approached
makes sense. On the other hand, if psychiatric conditions are not really
diseases, then it is hard to justify thinking about them from a medical
perspective.

There is a very large literature dealing with what we mean by disease.
Much of this literature is unsatisfactory because it wrestles with different
definitions of disease according to the biases of the authors. With regard
to psychiatric conditions, if the author is sympathetic to the idea that
they ought to be assigned to the responsibility of physicians, a definition

of disease is proposed that will include all or at least most psychiatric disorders. If the author is biased in the opposite direction, the definition will exclude all or most psychiatric problems.

I have argued elsewhere that it is not useful to approach this important question by struggling with the fundamental definition of disease because disease is a very general concept and one subject to change as medical knowledge advances (Guze 1970a). The same is true for concepts like disorder or illness. For most purposes, these terms are interchangeable. Scadding (1990) has also argued against the appropriateness of a definition of "disease-in-general." He refers to Popper's position against "essentialist" definitions that "have no place in science." Instead, Scadding argues that "in medical discourse, the name of a disease refers to the sum of the abnormal phenomena displayed by a group of living organisms in association with a specified common characteristic, or set of characteristics, by which they differ from the norm of their species in such a way as to place them at a biological disadvantage."

The idea of disease in general is an elusive concept, perhaps like evil or good. Such concepts can be defined, but the definitions rarely prove to be clear and free of qualifications or even contradictions. They nearly always leave room for disagreements as to which specific conditions ought to be included or excluded. Furthermore, as the definitions are put into use, it often becomes clear that they fail to take into consideration new knowledge or special circumstances that require modifications in the basic concept.

Turning to standard dictionaries, both general and medical, we find that their definitions of concepts like disease do not permit an easy decision about what to include under the category and, equally important, what to exclude. The *Oxford English Dictionary* (2nd edition, 1989) defines disease as "1a. Absence of ease; uneasiness, discomfort; inconvenience, annoyance; disquiet, disturbance; trouble. 1b. A cause of discomfort or distress; a trouble, an annoyance, a grievance. *Obs.* 2. A condition of the body, or of some part or organ of the body, in which its functions are disturbed or deranged; a morbid physical condition; a departure from the state of health, especially when caused by structural change. 2a. The condition of being (more or less seriously) out of health; illness, sickness. 2b. An individual case or instance of such a condition; an illness, ailment, malady, disorder. 2c. Any one of the various kinds of such conditions; a species of disorder or ailment, exhibiting special symptoms or affecting a special organ."

The *American Heritage Dictionary of the English Language* (1969) defines disease as "1. An abnormal condition of the organism or part, especially as a consequence of infection, inherent weakness, or environmental stress, that impairs normal physiological functioning. 2. A condition or tendency, as of society, regarded as abnormal or pernicious. 3. Obsolete. Lack of ease."

Webster's New Collegiate Dictionary (1963) defines it as "an impairment of the normal state of the living animal or plant body that affects the performance of the vital functions." It offers "sickness" as a synonym.

Dorland's Illustrated Medical Dictionary (27th edition, 1988) defines disease as "any deviation from or interruption of the normal structure or function of any part, organ, or system (or combination thereof) of the body that is manifested by a characteristic set of symptoms and signs and whose etiology, pathology, and prognosis may be known or unknown."

Stedman's Medical Dictionary (22nd edition, 1972) defines it as "Morbus; illness; sickness; an interruption or perversion of function of any of the organs; a morbid change in any of the tissues, or an abnormal state of the body as a whole, continuing for a longer or shorter period." Finally, *Webster's New Dictionary of Synonyms* (1968) offers the following synonyms: "affection, ailment, malady, complaint, and distemper."

These definitions indicate clearly that the term disease does not carry very specific meaning. It may refer to a wide variety of conditions, so that, in fact, "any condition associated with discomfort, pain, disability, death, or an increased liability to these states, *regarded by physicians and the public as properly the responsibility of the medical profession*, may be considered a disease" (Guze, 1970a). If follows, therefore, that whether a condition is regarded as a disease, and hence to be dealt with medically, is determined by many factors, social, economic, biologic, and so on. There is a similarity here with Scadding's view that the concept of disease involves the notion of biological disadvantage.

It is apparent that many illnesses have passed through transitions in the way they have been regarded. Epilepsy, mania, and other forms of

psychosis are examples of a shift from a magical or theological orientation to a medical one. Similar (though secular) shifts seem to be taking
place currently with regard to alcoholism and some personality disorders, especially antisocial personality. The scope of medical interest,
responsibility, and competence are evolving and changing as medical
knowledge grows and as medicine is being subjected to many complex
social, economic, and political forces.

At about the time I was struggling with this problem of the definition
of disease, and coming to the conclusions just enunciated, the American Psychiatric Association conducted a mail poll to determine the views
of its members concerning whether or not homosexuality should be
classified as a psychiatric disorder. Most of those who responded were
opposed. This led to appropriate changes in the official classification of
psychiatric disorders. A more vivid example of my thesis about the definition of disease could not have been anticipated. Over a short period
of time, homosexuality was regarded by physicians primarily as a moral
problem (a sin), then primarily as a medical problem (a psychiatric disorder), and "finally" as simply an alternate form of sexual orientation,
requiring no intervention.

The direction of this last shift concerning homosexuality was un-
usual, however. Most changes have been toward a medical view, mainly
because of new data, new insights about possible causal factors, including genetic ones, or new treatments. *Nevertheless, it seems obvious that
a given profession's claim for assuming any jurisdiction will be justified
only by demonstrating that the profession can help understand or man-
age a given condition.* In general, it seems better if these issues are not
settled solely by political action or debate. One can at least hope that
systematic data from appropriate research will contribute to enlightened
political discussions and thus to wise decisions.

Most of us who adhere to the medical model believe that the fullest
understanding of human health and illness, including psychiatric conditions, will depend increasingly on growing knowledge in biology, conceptualized very broadly. This will be more completely discussed later,
but the explicit as well as intuitive recognition of this explains the re-
definition of many personal and social problems into concerns of medicine.

Definitions of disease provide a background against which to consider efforts to develop a definition that is more specific (Guze 1978a). A sharply limited definition of disease that many people intuitively hold requires the presence of consistent anatomical changes in one or another body systems or evidence of a deviation from the normal in some biochemical or physiological process. This would certainly exclude most if not all psychiatric conditions as they are understood today.

However, this definition would also exclude certain nonpsychiatric conditions that all physicians recognize as diseases. High blood pressure is a good example because it is typically present for years without symptoms or disability and without consistent anatomical or biochemical changes. In addition, it is still not completely settled whether high blood pressure usually represents just the upper end of a normal distribution of blood pressures or rather some as yet unrecognized abnormality in the regulation of blood pressure. In addition, it is possible that some cases are manifestations of a normal distribution of blood pressure while others represent certain specific deviations in regulation. Despite these ambiguities about how high blood pressure fits into the definition of disease, all physicians recognize its role in the pathogenesis of a variety of cardiovascular conditions and its adverse effects on morbidity and mortality, and no one argues that high blood pressure ought not to be considered a disease.

Cardiac dysrhythmias present similar problems. These disorders in cardiac function often occur in the absence of recognizable anatomical or biochemical abnormalities in the heart, though they are frequently seen as complications of gross heart disease as well. Even when no satisfactory explanation for the abnormal heart rhythm is available, it may be associated with great fear and disability and it may be life-threatening.

Another example of what can happen when too narrow a definition of disease is applied may be seen in epilepsy. In the great majority of cases, consistent neuropathological changes cannot be detected. Epilepsy was as difficult to define and classify before the electrical activity of the brain could be measured by the electroencephalograph (EEG) as many psychiatric disorders are today. But who would argue that it became a disease only after the EEG was developed?

Formerly, epilepsy represented what some even today call a "functional" disorder. This, too, is an ambiguous concept, since all disorders, illnesses, or diseases are manifestations of disordered function. Yet the term functional is typically used as a substitute for psychological or psychiatric, and in most cases where it is applied, little or nothing is known about which functions are disturbed.

Among conditions most physicians and most laypersons regard as medical are many states for which consistent anatomical changes have not yet been demonstrated (Guze 1978b). These states may sometimes be manifestations of being at one or the other end of a normal distribution; at other times, they are manifestations of a qualitative deviation in some bodily process. Other states may indicate only an increased vulnerability to manifest disorder if exposed to specific environmental circumstances. Some are encountered only infrequently; others may occur in most of the population. Some may lead to severe disability; others only to minimal handicap; and a few may never cause difficulty if treated.

What ought we to conclude from these observations? The concept of disease in general is a convention, a metaphorical concept. Because of limited and imperfect knowledge, all definitions of disease are ambiguous, and the limits of the concept cannot be sharply defined. It is to be expected that new understanding will affect these limits (Guze 1978a). Furthermore, "it may be said that there is no such thing as disease; there are only diseases. The concept of disease may be a 'myth.' But, if so, it is a myth when applied to all medical conditions and not just when applied to psychiatric disorders" (Guze 1978b).

While disease as a general concept is vague and inherently ambiguous and subject to change, it is possible to achieve greater specificity, precision, and concreteness in defining individual conditions. Thus, lobar pneumonia, gout, paroxysmal atrial tachycardia, and essential hypertension can be defined so that physicians may share their experiences, teach, evaluate treatment, and look for causes, all independent of their ability to reach agreement about the definition of disease in general (Guze 1978a). The same can be said about schizophrenia, mania, obsessional disorder, and other psychiatric conditions.

If repeated and extensive efforts have failed to define disease so as to settle the question as to whether psychiatric conditions are properly classified as medical, what is meant by proposing that the medical model be the basis for approaching psychiatric conditions? Psychiatrists can utilize the concepts and methods derived from general medical experience in thinking about diagnosing and treating patients who are suffering from psychiatric disorders.

Diagnosis and the Medical Model

A long accepted assumption in medicine and now a central feature of the medical model is that illnesses come in many different forms. And it has been further assumed that these different forms typically reflect differences in causal factors, pathophysiology, epidemiology, and response to interventions. These assumptions point the direction for medical strategies—in general medicine and in psychiatry. Deciding what is wrong with the patient is obviously the basic step in clinical medicine. The medical term for this activity and for its result is diagnosis. Making a diagnosis involves classifying the illness.

Physicians have learned over the centuries that the manifestations of illness are not random. They have also come to understand that certain manifestations of illness often occur together and reflect disturbances involving different organs or even different parts of organs. Physicians recognize that certain combinations of symptoms and signs point to heart disease, for instance, while other symptoms and signs point to liver disease, and so on. Some manifestations typically reflect disturbances of the entire body or person: fever, malaise, and fatigue. Differential diagnosis refers to the essential activity in which the physician considers the diagnostic possibilities associated with the particular pattern of manifestations in a given patient.

Those who apply the medical model to psychiatric conditions have the same underlying assumptions that have served physicians in the rest of medicine. We assume that there are many different kinds of psychiatric disorders and that ultimately these different disorders will also turn out to arise from different causes and have different pathophysiologic mechanisms. We also assume that these different disorders will have different epidemiologic characteristics and that they will respond differently to different interventions. In fact, these assumptions have already been supported by the findings from numerous studies carried out in many different countries (Goodwin and Guze 1989).

Thus, psychiatrists must learn to recognize the many different kinds of psychiatric conditions, appreciate the elements of differential diagnosis, study the clinical course and outcome of the various disorders, realize their differential response to various different treatments, and understand their different epidemiologic characteristics. This is not different from what physicians must learn about medical disorders.

There is another fundamental assumption underlying modern medical thinking that has its counterpart in the application of the medical model to psychiatry. All physicians believe that improvements in diagnosis and treatment will depend to a large degree on advances in basic biomedical knowledge. The more we learn about the body's development, structure, and function, at all levels, from the integrative activity of the whole body to cellular and molecular processes, the more likely we are to become effective in understanding, treating, and preventing disease. For psychiatry, of course, this assumption includes special emphasis on advances in understanding the brain.

The essential assumptions involved in applying the medical model to psychiatric conditions are really quite simple. The first is that psychiatric disorders come in a rich variety of different states with all the implications noted above. The second assumption is that advances in neuroscience will contribute very importantly to improved understanding and treatment of such disorders.

The medical model is less concerned with definitions of disease and more with strategies for thinking about, studying, and taking care of sick people. It provides a framework for teaching, research, and clinical practice that has supported the advances made in general medicine; it will do the same for psychiatry. The medical model also offers a basis for important policy decisions that must be made about psychiatric disorders, including organizational, legal, and economic ones. Thus, questions concerning the roles of psychiatrists versus other mental health practitioners, the nature of appropriate training for psychiatric practice, access to hospital privileges and the right to prescribe medications, the significance of psychiatric conditions under the law, involuntary hospitalization, medical insurance coverage for psychiatric conditions, and many more will be answered differently depending upon one's adherence to the medical model. These questions will be discussed further later in the book.

Other Models: Sociocultural

The medical model, of course, is not without rivals in psychiatry. There are three broad alternative approaches that can be characterized most simply as sociocultural, psychodynamic, and behaviorist.

The sociocultural model assumes that psychiatric conditions simply represent understandable reactions to stressful or other meaningful circumstances in the psychosocial environment, past or present. Cultural and economic forces are typically viewed as crucial variables in explaining psychiatric conditions. The role of interindividual differences between people—other than those attributable to previous differences in psychosocially meaningful life experiences—is minimized. Thus, genetic and other differences are largely ignored. This view of psychiatric disorder may be summarized—without too much distortion—by the assertion that such conditions are the result of people being mistreated by their families, cultures, or social and political systems.

Often, though not always, associated with this model is a tendency to accept what has been called "labeling theory" about psychiatric conditions. This theory holds that there is little or no reason to believe in the validity of psychiatric disorders. It argues instead that psychiatric diagnoses are simply "labels" used by psychiatrists to provide a way for society to control social or political deviants and that these labels stigmatize the individuals.

Of course, the widely recognized abuse of psychiatric practice by some Nazi and Soviet psychiatrists for ideological and political purposes indicates that psychiatry, like all other institutions in society, may be perverted by totalitarian political systems. Even though psychiatric diagnoses have been used to justify political repression this does not mean, however, that there is no validity to psychiatric illnesses.

Labeling theorists do not argue simply that there may be negative aspects of any psychiatric diagnosis or that psychiatry may be abused for political purposes, but that a psychiatric diagnosis carries no specific information and that the diagnostic process serves only for social control. Schizophrenia is a common example.

In one often cited study, psychiatrists were tricked into hospitalizing, as possible schizophrenics, individuals who had been coached to present themselves with complaints of vague auditory hallucinations (Rosenhan

1973). Extensive criticism of this study and its conclusions has been published, based primarily on analyses of what actually took place, but insufficient emphasis has been paid to one overriding defect in the author's reasoning.

The author's essential argument is that the failure or inability of the psychiatrists to recognize that their patients were imposters proves that schizophrenia does not exist. Its fallacy is clear. Many individuals gain admission to hospitals by faking chest pains, various "spells," bleeding, or other striking symptoms. Such individuals are often discharged after appropriate study with diagnoses such as suspected coronary artery disease, suspected epilepsy, or suspected peptic ulcer. The fact that such patients are able to puzzle and sometimes deceive physicians would certainly not be taken as evidence that there is no such thing as coronary artery disease, epilepsy, or peptic ulcer disease (Guze and Helzer 1985).

In fact, the Munchausen syndrome is well known to physicians; individuals sometimes present themselves to doctors with factitious manifestations of illness or with false histories suggesting serious illnesses. In every branch of medicine, physicians rely on the reports of patients concerning their experiences of illness. If a patient is determined to misslead the physician, he or she will succeed on occasion, at least partially. Sometimes the physician is not sure what to make of the patient's story, especially when it proves inconsistent with the physician's examination or with laboratory findings.

Not rarely, the physician may even wonder about the patient's veracity, but most physicians are properly reluctant to conclude that a patient is faking until they have become well acquainted with him or her. Under such circumstances, it is not surprising that a physician will label the case as "suspected. . . ." Few would conclude from this, however, that physicians are unable to make valid diagnoses or that other patients do not present with similar complaints on the basis of real illnesses.

I would not argue that diagnoses are free from all sorts of psychological and social consequences. Quite the contrary: patients with all kinds of illnesses, including syphilis, leprosy, cancer, many psychiatric conditions, and of course, now AIDS, experience many adverse personal and social responses to their medically labelled condition. Very often, these responses may be as burdensome as the illness itself; sometimes, they are even worse than the illness.

It is important, however, to distinguish between the condition itself and the name applied to it. For example, not using the diagnosis of AIDS would not eliminate the disease, not would it eliminate all of the disease's social consequences. Even if we were to change the nomenclature of disorders so that they were all designated by numbers, people would soon learn that diagnosis "4567" carried undesirable implications and it would lead to the same social complications as the previous term.

This point is as applicable to psychiatric as to medical disorders. Mental illnesses can be every bit as painful, disabling, and frightening as many other medical conditions, and they often involve increased mortality as well.

Furthermore, denying the validity of psychiatric conditions sends a message to their victims and their families that is harmful and cruel. It says that the patients and their families are not entitled to the same consideration, sympathy, and compassion that our society rightfully grants to sick people. Nearly all of us who spend our lives working with psychiatric patients and their families consider the "labeling theory" fundamentally ludicrous. Any one with an open mind who spent a day on the wards of a psychiatric hospital talking to and observing patients and meeting their relatives would quickly be disabused of the notion.

Yet sociocultural and other environmental factors may be very important in the etiology and course of many psychiatric conditions (see Chapters 4 and 5). Psychiatric illnesses, like all illnesses, are most comprehensively conceptualized within a broad epidemiological framework, where health and disease are seen as varying aspects of the organism's efforts to adapt to its environmental circumstances and history.

Other Models: Psychodynamic

The second broad alternative to the medical model is the psychodynamic model, which in its most highly developed form is known as psychoanalysis. There are many different variations on this model, but they all are derivatives of Freud's basic ideas.

To start with, psychoanalysis offers one of the most comprehensive theories of human psychological development—one of its most attractive features. But at the same time it is a great weakness because the theory is exposed to such a wide range of criticisms, by purporting to explain all mental functions in health and disease. Psychoanalysis has proposed the same fundamental concepts and explanations for all psychiatric conditions, all personality disorders, many so-called psychosomatic conditions, accidents, conflicts, and war. Any theory that attempts to explain such a wide range of clinical, personal, and social problems raises serious questions. Is the theory so general that it can account for so much by really saying very little that is truly valid? Or does the theory have little to do with the conditions it purports to explain because it deals with nonspecific issues that are not highly correlated with the problems of concern?

In psychoanalytic theory, as in many other theories of human psychology, infancy and childhood are regarded as critical periods in the individual's development. As the individual matures and works at solving the specific challenges and tasks associated with different levels of development, certain unconscious memories or symbols of these experiences are formed that will play determinative roles in the rest of the individual's life. These unconscious residues of experience are seen as the *root causes* of all psychopathology. In fact, the theory uses these same unconscious residues to explain *all* human behavior. Examples of such unconscious residues of experience are "hatred of the introjected mother figure," "castration fear," "penis envy," "latent homosexuality," "conficts with authority figures," "Oedipus conflict," and so on.

The theory is built upon the belief that these unconscious memories or residues cannot be accepted by the individual because of their content, which is generally sexual or aggressive. As a result, the individual uses inherent psychological mechanisms of defense (repression, denial, projection, sublimation, etc.) to keep the content from consciousness. These defense mechanisms are not perfect, allowing manifestations of the unconscious residues of experience to occur in the form of dreams, slips of the tongue, responses to certain projective psychological tests, free associations, and a wide array of symptoms and illnesses.

Psychodynamic theories have depended very greatly upon two fundamental, related axioms or assumptions. The first is that psychological responses must be the result of psychological causes; this is sometimes referred to as "psychological determinism" (Gabbard 1990b, Sulloway 1979). The second, and derivative of the first, is that psychopathology is best viewed as fulfilling some unconscious psychological purpose; this is sometimes expressed by the question "Why did this patient need to express this symptom?" or "What is the advantage to the patient of this

symptom?" Not all psychoanalysts accept these axioms with equal enthusiasm (Edelson 1988), but these axioms have been important elements in the history and development of psychoanalytic theory. Thus,
psychodynamic theory provides no truly satisfactory way to deal with
psychological responses that are clearly caused by some chemical or
physiological alteration.

It is not that psychodynamic practitioners cannot understand that some
psychopathological manifestations are the result of brain abnormalities,
but psychoanalytic theory, *per se*, provides no basis for distinguishing
between such different circumstances, except to take note of the presence or absence of a *recognizable or known alteration in the patient's
brain*.

Some years ago, Dr. John Whitehorn, a professor of psychiatry at
Johns Hopkins, raised the same point in a metaphorical way (Whitehorn 1952). Discussing the psychodynamics of schizophrenia, he noted
that the "ready disclosure of . . . psychoanalytically 'symbolic' material
may be compared to the disclosure of intimate housekeeping details by
the collapse of the facade of a bombed apartment house. Many schizophrenic patients happen, by reason of their particular form of reaction,
to drop the social facade maintained so meticulously by ordinary mor-
tals."

Whitehorn's metaphor is an excellent one, and it should be kept in
mind when considering many such psychodynamic formulations. His
argument suggests vividly how difficult it is to determine the causal
relationship, *if any*, between an overt clinical disorder and various psychodynamic issues. Thus, if one considers the possibility that many, if
not most, psychiatric disorders result from some variation in brain function, the possibility clearly arises that the patient's "disclosures" may not
be specific to the disorder under study.

Initially, Freud seemed interested in the possibility that there might
be a certain regularity or specificity between the particular unconscious
nexus of the problems and forces he believed he was uncovering and
the overt clinical manifestations of the patient's disorder (Sulloway 1979).
He referred to this question as the "choice of the neurosis," including
under neurosis all sorts of clinical conditions such as delusions and
hallucinations and the full panoply of symptoms of psychiatric illness.

The scientific question may be encapsulated by asking: why did this
patient develop the particular presenting clinical problem or disorder

rather than a different set of problems or disorders? After his early attention to this important matter, Freud gradually seemed to lose interest in
the question of specificity, and his disciples tended to ignore it. This
marked a turning point of psychoanalytic theory away from the medical
model.

In turning away from the question of specificity, psychoanalysis avoided
dealing with the challenging questions: If all individuals experience the
difficulties of early development leading to unresolved unconscious forces
constantly struggling for expression, why do some develop psychoses
while others develop recurrent depressions or mania and still others fail
to develop any significant psychopathology? It avoided any need to show
that the uncovered unconscious residues of experience differed between
individuals with different clinical conditions.

Psychoanalysis seems to view all psychiatric disorders as a medley of
different manifestations, such as hallucinations, delusions, anxiety,
depression, obsessions, and so on. Any given illness in a particular individual at a specific time will be a mixture of such features. Sometimes
delusions will be prominent; at other times obsessions will dominate the
clinical picture and so forth. Pursuing this approach, one is less likely
to be interested in the particular mixture of signs and symptoms; instead, one is concerned primarily with the putative underlying, unconscious phenomena. This implies rejection of the fundamental assumption of the medical model that the differences and similarities seen among
different individual patients are *major* clues to understanding etiology
and ultimately to effective intervention.

Freud's early approach was conditioned by his interest in the biological thinking of his day (Sulloway 1979). Though somewhat ambigu-
ously and inconsistently, he often emphasized that his theory was really
an attempt to provide a biological base to psychology. He absorbed con-
temporary ideas about instincts, but the importance of human biological variability and its association with genetic variability were not yet
broadly assimilated into the biomedical perspectives of his time, even
though Darwin's ideas were widely known and apparently influenced
Freud's thinking (Sulloway 1979).

Psychoanalysis and other psychodynamic approaches, to this day, have
not yet integrated into their psychodynamic theories modern insights
and knowledge from epidemiology, genetics, and neurobiology. It is not
so much that they deny the validity of the findings from these sciences

as that they do not seem to know how these new insights would alter the original theories. By continuing to explain the etiology and patho-genesis of such disorders as schizophrenia, mania, obsessional disorder, and antisocial personality according to the same basic formulations, psy-choanalysis fails to take into account evidence from many different stud-ies all over the world that these conditions have different epidemiologic characteristics, different genetic patterns, and different responses to dif-ferent pharmacologic treatments (Goodwin and Guze 1989).

Other Models: Behaviorism

The third alternative to the medical model for psychiatry is behavior-ism. The essential feature of this approach is emphasizing overt, objec-tive behavior, including physiological measurements, while, at the same time, rejecting the scientific value of inner psychological states for pur-poses of studying cause and effect. B.F. Skinner put it as follows: "Nar-rowly considered . . . the special province of psychology may be taken to be the description of the behavior of the individual as a whole and the explanation of that behavior in terms of environmental factors and conditions. More specifically, psychology is concerned with recording and measuring human behavior and its various aspects, and with relat-ing the quantities so measured to variables in the past and current en-vironment. . . . Mental disease appears to refer to modes of behavior which are troublesome or dangerous either to the individual himself or to others" (Skinner 1959, page 195).

J.V. Brady argued similarly: "This is not to say that the problems associated with consciousness or the phenomenal world are uninterest-ing or unimportant. Indeed, philosophers and theologians, among oth-ers, have been grappling with the mysteries of mental life since time immemorial. And while it is evident that mental processes cannot be denied experientially, their conceptual status as more than collateral effects (i.e., epiphenomena) of complex brain-behavior interactions lacks empirical support. . . . Among the more obvious problems raised by such mentalistic approaches to an appiled branch of medical science [referring to psychiatry generally] is their definition in terms of abstrac-tions that have neither weight, extension, nor other physical proper-ties."

Brady continues: "Metaphorical (and in some prominent instances allegorical) referents replace operational language, diverting attention from confrontable realities and encouraging appeals to explanatory fictions. Mental processes are represented as causal agents, and the view of 'autonomous man' that emerges is inimical to the methods of procedure and the rules of evidence that characterize the tradition of natural science—a tradition that has proven particularly fruitful in other areas of applied biology and in the general conduct of human affairs" (Brady 1988).

Professor Alexander Rosenberg, a philosopher of science and especially of social science, under which he specifically includes psychology, in a careful and balanced discussion of behaviorism, points out (Rosenberg 1988, page 53) that it argues that "for purposes of psychology . . . we don't need the hypothesis that people have minds—mental states like belief and desire, sensations like pain or colors. . . . Rather it declares that questions about the mind are irrelevant on the following grounds: First, human behavior can be explained without appeal to the mind; second, it cannot be explained by such appeals; and third, questions about the mind are themselves unanswerable in any case. Therefore, for purposes of science, we might as well just ignore the mind."

In essence, behaviorism denies the value of devoting much attention to the mental activities of patients and attributing to these mental experiences any causal effects. Behaviorists are willing to make place for what the patient says, but they do not appear to be willing to differentiate between what the patient subjectively experiences and what is reported. This is like not recognizing the difference between a map and the place being described. All of us know that we repeatedly experience many thoughts and feelings without giving voice to them so that others can know about them too. This shows that the subjective experience and its overt expression are not the same thing even if they often overlap. We all also know that it is impossible to deny the possibility that the subjective experience can have important causal effects.

With very few exceptions, psychiatrists accept the validity of subjective experience, our own as well as that of our patients. We recognize in addition that for the most part clinical psychiatry focuses on such experience. We understand that we learn about such experiences from what the patient tells us and that it is not always easy to grasp fully and understand what the patient is experiencing. We also know that some patients have great difficulty in articulating what they feel. And sadly, we have learned that some patients sometimes deliberately mislead us.

Nevertheless, we see little merit in throwing away the usefulness of subjective experience in our efforts to understand and help our patients. In this, we are once again following the medical model: physicians have always paid attention to the patient's complaints as valuable, and often essential, guides to diagnosis.

There are many psychiatric patients whose overt behavior is not particularly remarkable, except for their reports of their subjective experiences. If a patient complains of certain obsessions, such as recurrent and disturbing ideas or impulses of a sexual or religious nature, which cannot be controlled, we would run the risk of appearing arrogant to insist that they are unimportant unless manifested in the patient's behavior. If a patient reports that he or she has been suffering from a long period of depression that includes delusional ideas of sinfulness and guilt and that he or she has considered suicide, it would be foolish to ignore the risk. Additionally, it seems unwise to ignore the possibility that the suicide attempt may have been at least partly the result of the depression. Or if the patient describes a complicated delusional system with well-developed paranoid features and offers these fears as the motive for killing a neighbor, would it be wise to reject categorically this possibility with the argument that it is based upon an "explanatory fiction" of an "autonomous man"? Behaviorism has been extremely useful in describing the basis for some human behavior as an experimental paradigm, but it is too limited a foundation for the structure of clinical psychiatry.

Yet it is certainly true that we cannot determine whether or not we all are experiencing the same thing when we use the same words to describe subjective experiences. For some people, this means that a truly scientific approach to such experiences is not possible, so that they fall back on some version of behaviorism. But the same concern can be raised about the words we use to describe more objective experiences, like past overt behavior. How can we ever know that we are all using particular descriptive words in the same way? And if this too is beyond scientific study, where do we find ourselves?

It seems evident that we must be aware of the problems such questions raise, but still proceed to establish the strongest validity possible for both the subjective experiences and the descriptions of them through scientific efforts to build up meaning within a network of consistent correlations and causal experimental contexts. Complete certainty may not be achievable, but useful knowledge may, nevertheless, be attained.

In a recent book, H. Damasio and A.R. Damasio (1989), two neurologists at the University of Iowa interested in cognitive science, argue that there is a "shift away from the behaviorist model of psychology, which had made the relationship between stimuli and response the only legitimate object of study and treated mind and brain as a black box. In its place, a cognitive model that reinstates the reality of mental phenomena and makes nonverbal as well as verbal representations a valid focus of psychological inquiry has gained acceptance. . . . In the new approach, subjects' behavioral responses are not just linked to the stimuli that eventually triggered them, but are connected to mind processes and representations that handled the stimulus and generated the responses according to some mechanism. The investigators no longer shy away from formulating hypotheses about those mechanisms and attempting to test their validity, indirectly, by measuring external responses."

2

Research Implications of the Medical Model

Scientific Strategies

What is the most appropriate scientific strategy for applying the medical model to research on psychiatric disorders? Here again, turning to experience in the rest of medicine offers valuable instruction. Over the years, medical research has involved two broad paths. The first has been to account for the incidence, prevalence, and varied manifestations of illnesses in terms of environmental and demographic factors. These include geography, climate, culture, socioeconomic status, family characteristics, interpersonal relationships, nutrition, infectious agents, toxic chemicals, occupation, age, sex, education, and treatment. The concepts and methods for this kind of research have evolved primarily from the fields of epidemiology and biostatistics.

The second broad path of medical research has been to account for the clinical manifestations of disease in terms of the structure and function of the body at many different levels, from that of the organ system to that of cellular and molecular processes. The research concepts and techniques for this kind of investigation have evolved from modern biological laboratory science.

These two dimensions of scientific research come together at the clinical level, where physicians must consider the history of the patient's illness, including detailed consideration of specific symptoms and complaints, and the results of physical and mental status examinations, including findings from radiographic and other imaging techniques, and from standard diagnostic laboratory tests, as well as psychological tests. The concepts and methods used at the clinical level derive from laboratory science, epidemiology, and biostatistics.

Applying the medical model to psychiatric conditions means that these same scientific paths and strategies are appropriate for research dealing with psychiatric concerns. These approaches provide appropriate places for all the possibly relevant factors associated with psychiatric illness that have been suggested by psychiatrists and other mental health professionals. The epidemiologic path of investigation permits the study and measurement of all sorts of cultural, socioeconomic, and familial factors that have been proposed as causal or modifying factors in such illness. The clinical level offers full opportunity to study and think about the patient's subjective experiences, coping skills, communications, and expectations. The laboratory path obviously includes the study of anatomical, physiological, and chemical changes associated with illness. All three may be involved in studies of treatment. The medical model thus excludes no conceptual or methodological approach to research or practice suggested by those experienced in the field.

This is an important point to emphasize because many assume that the medical model excludes from consideration the patient's psychosocial environment and subjective experiences. Some even go so far as to equate the medical model with an exclusive focus on body chemistry and the prescribing of psychoactive drugs.

Nothing could be more incorrect. All physicians must consider all aspects of the patient's environment to understand fully the etiology of illness and optimize treatment programs (Reiss et al. 1991). Epidemiological studies have been indispensable in the evolution of our understanding of many clinical conditions, from coronary artery disease to alcoholism. Such studies have identified very important factors that contribute to the risk of these two conditions, as well as many others. It has been through epidemiological investigations that the roles of culture, sex, race, age, diet, occupation, family illness patterns, and much else, have been established for many different disorders.

Of course, to establish the significance of any environmental factor in disease requires careful, controlled, and repeated studies, just as it does with physiological or genetic factors (Guze 1970a, Guze and Helzer 1985). Plausibility is not enough; systematic and controlled data are necessary.

That psychiatric disturbances arise from the social and psychological environment appears to be so plausible that hypotheses often are not critically examined. It is evident that everyone is influenced greatly by the social environment: language, customs, religion, politics, and ethics are acquired from this environment. Culture so profoundly shapes and influences our ideas, attitudes, and behavior that we assume it must also shape personality and temperament.

Yet to say this is not very useful; we need to know *which* social factors, under *which* circumstances, predispose to *which* personality traits or psychiatric disturbance. In other words, specific associations need to be established before useful causal connections between social environment and psychopathology can be established. We must show that a given psychiatric condition results from either more or less of a given environmental influence, or that it results from a particular kind of environmental influence (Guze 1970a). These requirements are not different from those applied to hypotheses concerning cellular or molecular etiologies for psychiatric disorders, though psychosocial environmental influences are particularly difficult to quantify.

Pitfalls in Research: Selecting Subjects

Studies to test environmental hypotheses about psychopathology are plagued with difficulties. Biased selection of subjects, poorly selected controls, imprecision in defining or measuring life events or psychosocial stress, failure to take into consideration the great significance of the time interval between stress and illness, difficulty in distinguishing the causes of illness from the consequences of illness, and insufficient attention to the effect of observer bias are among the serious problems (Guze 1984).

In any study of the role of environmental psychological or social factors in disease, the investigator must select subjects in such a way as to exclude the possibility that the very factors being studied influence the likelihood of a subject's being selected. Social class, education, ethnicity, marital status, and occupation, for example, are associated with different risks of developing many disorders, including psychiatric ones, and these same factors can influence the likelihood that an individual will be selected for study. For example, neighborhoods, clinics, hospitals, individual private practices and workplaces vary greatly in the characteristics of their populations. To the extent that such different distributions of demographic characteristics exist and are not recognized and controlled for, erroneous conclusions can follow from the studies.

Similar concerns are necessary in the selection of controls as well.

Selecting controls from different streams of patients may result in observed differences that simply reflect biases in choosing physician or clinic, rather than differences truly related to the factors under study. As examples: choosing controls from a general medicine clinic for comparison with subjects from a psychosomatic medicine clinic or selecting controls from volunteers derived from hospital or medical school employees and staff for comparison with patients in such institutions may confound the effects of the variables under study with the effects of social class, education, sophistication, attitudes toward the study, and the already noted biases of patient selection (Guze 1984).

The ideal way to eliminate this problem is to carry out extensive, long-term epidemiological investigations in which the study population is selected so as to represent a true cross section of the population at large. This is a formidable undertaking. It necessitates a large number of subjects who are in good health and whose environments vary sufficiently to allow for appropriate comparison. The characteristics of the environment must be assessed *before* any of the subjects becomes ill, so as to remove any possibility of confounding the results by the effects of illness on the environment. Such confounding is clearly possible when an illness affects interpersonal relationships or work patterns, but illness can also lead to changes in living arrangements and even to moving to different climates.

Alvan Feinstein considered these problems deeply and has suggested a way to get around the practical difficulties in such prospective studies. He proposed what he calls follow-back studies in which the sample is identified after the illness has been recognized and then the records are searched in a systematic and controlled way for data bearing on the hypothesized causal factor (Feinstein 1967, Feinstein 1985). This strategy can work for hypotheses that deal with variables likely to be included in the records of the past. Unless this is true, however, it generally proves impossible to take advantage of this strategy.

To return to the population-based strategy, the sample must be followed to identify new cases of the condition being studied and correlate the incidence of these cases with the suspected environmental factors. If a long interval is necessary before the development of a significant number of new cases, this raises the question whether the environmental factors under study have changed during the interval. It is not surprising, therefore, that few such investigations have been undertaken.

Instead, investigators resort to more limited and potentially more biased samples and must carefully consider potentially confounding variables in selecting their subjects and their controls.

At the same time, there is no practical way to conduct an experimental study dealing with the etiological role of the long-term psychosocial environment in humans. Ethical and legal considerations prohibit the kind of unbiased, random assignment of individuals to experimental and control groups that is necessary but only feasible in animal studies. Even if it were possible to obtain sufficient volunteers, only short-term, highly focused experiments could be carried out.

Though it may be possible to study the effect of a relatively short-term exposure to a particular food or chemical agent or a circumscribed experience, such as social isolation in a controlled environment, it is not possible to study the effect of a persistent or recurrent psychosocial context, such as prolonged marital discord. At the same time, animal studies are problematic for the investigation of psychiatric disorders, at a minimum because of limitations in communication.

We are forced, therefore, to take advantage of "nature's experiments"—such as natural disasters, bereavement, unemployment—in which the selection biases already discussed so often prove to be major hurdles to valid conclusions. Further, because it is so hard to eliminate all biases, replicability of findings, especially when reported by different investigators, is extremely important since we can expect that the biases will not be the same in all studies and that they will therefore cancel out one another, leaving valid observations.

Pitfalls in Research: Defining Life Situations

Selecting subjects and controls is not the only problem. To define and ascertain life situations, life stresses, and psychosocial pressures is no less difficult. In general, there is comparatively little ambiguity about certain events: the death of a parent, injury in an automobile accident, an episode of pneumonia, giving birth to a child, losing a job, getting divorced, and so on. These allow greater precision than an argument with a parent, disappointment in one's career, or a sense of frustration and failure of communication with a spouse. It is clear that for some of these events, high degrees of reliability of ascertainment of cases are possible; for others, inconsistency of such ascertainment seems inescapable.

To make matters worse, even when two events appear to be causally related, it is not easy to be sure that the life event and the putative consequence under study are truly independent of one another, even in the case of parental death years before. For example, the death of a mother from breast cancer when a patient with asthma was a child suggests no obvious hidden connections increasing the likelihood that the two conditions (mother's cancer and child's asthma) might be associated. On the other hand, if the mother had committed suicide and depression was being studied in the child, it would certainly be desirable to consider the possibility that the mother and daughter suffered from the same illness and that an underlying shared genetic predisposition was at least partly responsible for the association between the mother's death and the patient's depression.

A similar relationship might be entertained if a parent died of a cancer known to be associated with alcoholism (e.g., cancer of the larynx) and the condition under study in the child is also known to be associated with alcoholism (e.g., suicide). Since alcoholism is known to be familial and probably genetic to some extent, the parent's cancer and the child's suicide could be related to an underlying predisposition to alcoholism.

The point being made is not that there cannot be causal connections between parental experiences and illness in their children, but that we need to take into consideration the possibility that the apparent connection may not be a direct causal one, but may be at least equally well explained by a less apparent alternative connection. Such alternative explanations are common when we set out to draw conclusions from experiments of nature. If we cannot accept at face value an apparent causal association between death of a parent and illness in an offspring it should be no surprise that associations between other life events and various disorders can be similarly confounded.

For example, divorce may not simply be a cause of illness, it may just as easily be the result of illness. Early manifestations of many serious disorders may include irritability, apathy, reduced sexual drive, and other behavior that could contribute to divorce as well as be intensified by divorce. This must be considered when an association between divorce and illnesses is found and causal relationships are suggested (Guze 1984).

An example from the recent literature offers additional insight as to why it is necessary to try to control for the possibility that life events or stresses might be conditioned by attributes of the individual who is subjected to these environmental forces (Champion 1990). Champion set out to study the relationship between social vulnerability and the occurence of severely threatening life events. Her work grew out of studies by Brown and Harris (1978) on the development of depression in women indicating that psychosocial vulnerability mediated between negative life events and the illness.

Brown and Harris proposed four vulnerability factors: lack of an intimate confiding relationship with a husband or boyfriend, lack of employment outside the home, three or more children aged less than fourteen at home, and loss of mother before the age of eleven. However, Champion found that only lack of intimacy proved to be consistent in other studies. The significance of the other three factors was not replicated. She emphasizes that the role of vulnerability in increasing the likelihood of severe events occurring in the first place had been largely unexplored. Her reanalysis of several published studies revealed that lack of intimacy was associated with an increased occurrence of adversity. She concludes that in research on links between life events and psychiatric disorder, it is important to look at causes of life events that may be due to the "person's internal characteristics," thus possibly setting up a circular causal process.

These findings indicate how difficult it may be to draw valid conclusions concerning causal connections involving social and other environment experiences and psychiatric disorder in nature's experiments. Paul Meehl, a highly respected psychologist and philosopher of science at the University of Minnesota, has put the problem faced by investigators pithily by noting that in "correlational research there arises a special problem for the social scientist from the empirical fact that 'everything is correlated with everything else, more or less'" (Meehl 1990). This may be too skeptical, but it emphasizes the problems faced in such research.

Pitfalls in Research: Timing of Illness and Stresses

A closely related issue has to do with determining when a particular illness began and establishing a time window during which it is reasonable to hypothesize that a particular experience or stress may have played an etiological role. This is a difficult thing to do with most illnesses, including nearly all psychiatric disorders, because it is often impossible to date the onset of the condition with confidence.

As an example, many patients with schizophrenia experience a variety of difficulties in school and interpersonal relationships for months or years before they show the typical psychotic features. Did the condition have its onset when the non-diagnostic manifestations appeared? While the answer is uncertain, it is likely that different environmental experiences and forces were operating at the two different points in time.

Another example may be seen in anxiety disorders. Many patients with this condition report childhood fears and behaviors. Should the onset be defined as the patient's age when the childhood fears started or when panic attacks first occurred? Again, reasonable arguments can be made for each time period, but different environmental circumstances are likely to be associated with the different ages.

Similar problems are encountered in general medicine. Episodes of angina pectoris, for instance, typically experienced first in middle-age, develop many years after coronary artery atherosclerosis begins to narrow the lumen of these vessels. While episodes of chest pain are usually precipitated by exertion or strong emotion, there is little evidence that these factors cause the atherosclerosis itself.

While it may be clinically useful to know that the exacerbation of certain symptoms is correlated with events that appear to have psychological significance to the patient, it is fundamentally more important, of course, to know whether these events correlate with the underlying pathogenetic process itself. The first kind of knowledge may help the patient reduce the frequency and severity of the symptoms, but it is the second kind of knowledge that leads to understanding of etiology and offers hope for cure or prevention.

This brings us naturally to questions about the kinds of events, stresses, or life situations that supposedly precipitate or aggravate clinical disorders: marriage, divorce, the birth of a child, getting a new job, losing a job, loss of relatives and friends, moving, disagreements with relatives or friends, and so on. These are a part of nearly everyone's life, just like physical activity, climatic change, growing older, and exposure to microorganisms and a variety of toxic substances. In other words, if illness is viewed as a manifestation of the individual's adaptation to his or her complex environment, we must ask: how can we tell if the apparent association between the life experience and the illness is significant?

If all of us have similar life experiences, and yet only some get sick during the period when they are having these experiences, how can we be sure that the experiences played any role in the illness? Obviously, we must look for different patterns of experiences between those who get sick and those who do not. And we must simultaneously look for particular vulnerabilities that increase the likelihood of illness in some or, *conversely*, strengths that decrease the likelihood in others. Such differential vulnerability could result from genetic differences, previous experiences at critical periods of development, previous illnesses, or a variety of concurrent traits. Unfortunately, there has been frustratingly little consistency in the findings from different studies.

Research Pitfalls: The Impact of Illness on Subjects

An important consideration needs to be introduced here: the problems inherent in interpreting the significance of patients' reports concerning their experiences, attitudes, emotions, and expectations. It is self-evident that such reports about inner feelings are difficult to weigh, and difficult to compare. Though it is not as widely recognized, they are also vulnerable to the effects of illness. Pain, suffering, disability, impending death, or the fear of these have an influence, however difficult it may be to define, on thinking, feeling, and remembering.

Psychiatrists have recognized for a long time, for example, that depression often profoundly colors a patient's perception of his or her life. Pessimism, hopelessness, self-criticism, and guilt—typical manifestations of depression—can and frequently do lead to severe distortion in the way one's past life and achievements, one's future prospects, and one's personal relationships are perceived. For example, a successful career or marriage, under the weight of severe depression, can be reinterpreted with great conviction as a failure. Sometimes the distortion may be severe enough to lead to frank delusions, with the patient regarding himself or herself as sinful or under the control of the devil.

Such distortions make it almost impossible to confirm any etiological hypotheses derived from the patient's introspection and communication by further exploration of these same processes. It is necessary to seek confirmation outside the patient's reports (Guze 1984).

Research Pitfalls: Sociological Analysis

We have focused so far mainly on the individual patient's microenvironment, which includes relations with family, friends, home and so on. Beyond this lies sociological analysis. For example, several studies have shown that the proportion of patients suffering from schizophrenia who are of low socioeconomic status is greater than would be expected if social class and schizophrenia were not related (Dunham 1965, Goldberg and Morrison 1963).

This increased prevalence of low socioeconomic status was taken to indicate that there is something associated with lower status that increases the risk for developing schizophrenia. If this were true, it would clearly represent a very important finding about the etiology of the disease and would suggest that schizophrenia might be prevented by improving factors associated with low socioeconomic status, such as poor education, nutrition, medical care, and housing.

There is a reverse explanation, however, that is known as "downward drift." Conventional measures of socioeconomic status, such as education, occupation, place of residence, and income, are themselves greatly influenced by the schizophrenic disorder. The more serious manifestations of schiziphrenia typically begin to appear in late adolescence or early adulthood. Full clinical manifestations usually develop in the late twenties and early thirties, the average age of first hospitalization. This means that schizophrenia characteristically starts to flourish at the time in life when advanced education and the beginnings of a career are usually taking place. Thus, the illness itself may at least partially account for low socioeconomic status (Dunham 1965, Goldberg and Morrison 1963, Guze 1970a).

That this is probably true may be concluded from the results of several studies comparing the socioeconomic status of the parents of schizophrenic patients with that of the general population. There were no significant differences, which indicate that schizophrenic patients are not more likely to come from lower socioeconomic backgrounds and that their socioeconomic status is more likely the consequence than the partial cause of the illness (Dunham 1965, Goldberg and Morrison 1963, Guze 1970a). There may be similar patterns in other psychiatric conditions that begin early in life and seriously interfere with education and work.

Another sociological question of concern to psychiatry involves reported differences in suicide rates in different countries and in different cities within a single country like the United States. These have suggested various cultural and social factors in suicide. A major obstacle to the correct interpretations of such reports is the considerable variation—between countries, between cities, and over time—in the way cases of suicide are ascertained. If coroners or medical examiners in one area are more reluctant than their counterparts in other locations to designate a case as a suicide and instead call it accidental death, no one should be surprised that different suicide rates will be reported from the several sites. The stigma attached to suicide as well as insurance considerations may play a role in this.

Research Pitfalls: Nonpsychosocial Studies

Similar problems are encountered in nonpsychosocial studies. Apparently significant discoveries about biochemical differences associated with particular psychiatric disorders, for instance, have often turned out to be the result of confounding variables related to certain aspects of the patient's treatments (Murphy et al. 1962). This may be the case with the changes found at autopsy in the brains of schizophrenic patients treated with neuroleptic drugs who died after many years of illness. Many such patients show an increase in the number of dopamine receptors in various areas of the brain. This is of great interest because of the "dopamine hypothesis" of schizophrenia, which postulates that the fundamental symptoms of schizophrenia are the result of an excess of dopamine in certain specific anatomical areas of the brain.

This hypothesis, in turn, stemmed from the observation that all or nearly all pharmacologic agents that are clinically effective in the treatment of schizophrenia block specific dopamine receptors (Snyder 1986). The difficulty arises, however, from the fact that it is now well established, from animal studies, that the administration of antipsychotic agents leads to a very prolonged increase in the number and density of dopamine receptors, almost certainly a compensatory phenomenon. Thus, it is difficult to tell whether the findings at autopsy result from the illness or the treatment, or both. Similar findings in patients *who apparently had never received drug treatment for schizophrenia* raise questions, however, about the representativeness of such patients. Very few patients suffering from schizophrenia today, at least in countries with developed, Western-style medical systems, escape antipsychotic drug treatment entirely, leading to uncertainty about possible conclusions when such patients are compared to the great majority who receive significant treatment with antipsychotic drugs.

Another example involves an amusing though sad psychosocial explanation for what had been regarded by some as a possible infectious phenomenon. For many years reports have been appearing that more schizophrenics are born during the winter and early spring than during other seasons (Boyd et al. 1986, Dalen 1975, Pulver et al. 1983). It had been suggested that this might be a clue to the identification of a cause of schizophrenia associated with the winter months, perhaps some respiratory or other infection.

In a brief letter to the editor about these reports, D.F. Dawson noted that "Both studies showed a significant excess of births in the first quarter of the year for people who later became schizophrenic. The excess was approximately 8% for January, February, March and April. . . . Both articles listed a number of explanations for this finding, but they seem to have missed the simplest and most plausible explanation.

"The schizophrenic patients in both studies were born between 1920 and 1955. During that period, a large number of schizophrenics of childbearing age were institutionalized. A schizophrenic psychosis at that time probably meant a mental hospital admission lasting from at least three months to two years. Although the sexual activity of hospitalized schizophrenics is probably less than that of the nonhospitalized population, it certainly is not nonexistent."

Dawson continued "Male and female patients were on different wards but were permitted ground privileges in good weather. It is well known to the staff of most mental hospitals that in the private area of the grounds a fair amount of sexual activity takes place in good weather. In such cases, given the distribution of diagnoses in hospitalized patients, at least one of the procreating adults, often both, would have had a schizophrenic disorder.

"The excess births of schizophrenic patients in January, February, March, and April could easily be accounted for by the offspring of only a small percentage of the thousands of hospitalized patients. If conception did indeed take place during the warm months (June, July, August, and September) then a transmission rate of only 3%–5% would account for the excess number of schizophrenics born the next winter and early spring" (Dawson 1978).

To determine whether or not this hypothesis is correct, it would need to be tested by a careful review of whatever data are available or by looking for new information that might have a bearing on the matter. For starters, it would be helpful to know the number of children born to schizophrenic women who had been hospitalized at the correct time for the conception to have taken place during hospitalization. Similarly, it would be useful to have evidence that the frequency of winter and early spring births declined among younger schizophrenics whose hospitalizations occurred after the period of lengthy hospitalizations was followed by the current practice of briefer admissions, which might have reduced the likelihood of sexual encounters in the hospital.

Another interpretation of the apparently increased winter births has been proposed, however, by M. S. Lewis (1989a, 1989b, 1990). He argues that the findings may simply be the result of errors in the design and interpretation of seasonal studies. He maintains that the findings "reflect the 'age of incidence' effect. Very simply, this is the consequence of the fact that individuals born in January are older than individuals born in October, for example, and thus have lived through a larger proportion of the age of risk for the disorder under study."

Some studies indicate a season-of-birth effect may also be seen in patients with bipolar affective disorder, depressive disorder, mental retardation, hysteria, cancer, and tuberculosis (Lewis 1989a, 1989b, 1990) and for patients with Alzheimer's dementia (Philpot et al. 1989). The same finding across so many different disorders prompted Lewis to suggest that it is "easier to believe that they (the various reports) all contain the same artifact than to believe that they all have a season-of-birth component involved in their incidence."

A lively debate persists about this interpretation. It is not clear yet which will prove to be a better explanation for the findings: a "season-of-birth" effect or an "age of incidence" effect. It also still needs to be considered whether the "age of incidence" effect could operate in the southern hemisphere, from which reports have also come concerning "season-of-birth" effects.

Dwelling on the pitfalls in many causal interpretations about the development of psychiatric disease is not to say that such interpretations are wrong. Rather it is to call attention to the risk of confounding variables, to underline how difficult it is to draw firm conclusions from research on the etiology of any condition, including psychiatric disorders (Feinstein 1967, 1985).

The special difficulties of psychiatry, it has seemed to me, require an even greater commitment to the skepticism inherent in the scientific methods that medicine generally has embraced. It is difficult to make valid observations and accurate measurements of psychiatric phenomena. Because objectivity is elusive and unintended error is so easy, greater care is needed than in many other fields. Knowing how easy it is to form erroneous opinions in dealing with psychological phenomena and how hard it can be to eliminate or reduce observer bias, more rather than less is required in the way of repeated, systematic, controlled studies (Guze 1970a).

Paradoxically, this attitude has been attacked in the name of humanitarianism. It has been asserted, or implied, that the demand for data, for controls, for placing the burden of proof on the affirmative, reveals a lack of interest in people. Observing that the effectiveness of a particular treatment is still in doubt has led to the charge that the skeptic is antitherapeutic. It has even been argued that teaching a skeptical viewpoint too vigorously is harmful to medical students and psychiatric residents because it weakens their self-confidence and faith in what they are doing, which will, in turn, impair their effectiveness as therapists.

If that were true, it would be a serious consideration, but there is *no* evidence that this happens. Scientific skepticism is in no way incompatible with compassion for the sick or disabled. On the contrary, it is often the strong desire to help patients that causes psychiatrists to be frustrated by the lack of definite knowledge about what really helps and what does not. Few things are more humane than the effective use of knowledge to relieve suffering. The discovery of a truly effective treatment or prevention for schizophrenia would benefit millions of sufferers and their families all over the world.

In recent years there has been much progress in research on psychiatric disorders and in the development of treatment methods. It is still true, however, that a disturbingly high percentage of the population suffers from a clinically significant psychiatric disorder, frequently associated with great discomfort and disability, and often of long duration, and that many others have milder or more transient disturbances. It is still true that "the importance of the field far outstrips the available knowledge . . . [and that] only a great deal of careful, sophisticated, toughminded research is likely to improve the situation" (Guze 1970a).

3

Diagnosis

How does the medical model shape the approach of the physician to an individual psychiatric patient? Diagnosis and differential diagnosis have been characteristic medical activities for centuries, and they are fundamental in psychiatry as well. Psychiatric illnesses, like all other types of medical disorders, comprise a great variety of different conditions. Because we assume that these different psychiatric conditions will turn out to be associated with different etiological factors, pathophysiologic mechanisms, clinical features, epidemiological characteristics, and responses to various interventions (Guze 1970a, 1977, 1978b), it is important to distinguish between them.

As knowledge grows, many changes will take place in the way psychiatric disorders are grouped. This will probably mean new divisions of what were previously thought to be unitary conditions and new combinations of what were considered separate and distinct disorders. These changes may come about because of new insights into etiology or pathogenesis or because of consistent differential responses to specific treatments in subsets of patients who are currently not distinguished from one another.

The likelihood of such changes occurring in the future, however, does not reduce the need for classifying illnesses in the present. Diagnosis is simply the medical term for the classification of illnesses, both the activity and the product. It is still hard to understand fully how it was possible for a generation of American psychiatrists as recently as fifteen years ago to argue seriously against the central importance of psychiatric diagnosis. With the publication, in 1980, of the third edition of the American Psychiatric Association's Diagnostic and Statistical Manual (DSM-III), however, the fundamental importance of psychiatric diagnosis was officially reaffirmed.

Diagnosis and Communication

A classification of illnesses is indispensable for communication between physicians, for comparing the experiences of different physicians, for teaching and training medical students and young physicians, for research, and for thinking about medical problems. Without a diagnostic classification, the usefulness of clinical experience becomes problematic. The value of clinical experience is based on the assumption that the current clinical problem shares crucial attributes with past clinical problems so that it may prove helpful to approach the current problem with concepts similar to those that seemed helpful in the past. Diagnosis refers to these shared crucial attributes. If similar phenomena differing in time or place have no dependable, valid, shared crucial attributes that we can describe, it is hard to see what we might mean by the value of experience.

A British psychiatrist, Robert Kendell (1975), in an excellent book on the role of diagnosis in psychiatry, put it very succinctly when he wrote that "the advantage of a classification is quite simply that it allows us to communicate."

It is obviously very important to determine whether a patient suffers from pneumonia, pulmonary infarction, congestive heart failure, or bronchogenic carcinoma, even though the presenting clinical features may sometimes be quite similar. It is just as important to determine *whether the patient suffers from anxiety neurosis, alcoholism, schizophrenia, or hysteria, even though the presenting clinical pictures may again be similar* (Guze 1978a). The reason of course is that the different conditions require different treatment and have different prognoses.

The medical model is not based upon any assumptions about etiology. It can accept social and psychological events as causes just as well as physical and chemical events. It can accept single causes or multiple causes. It can even be applied when the etiology is unknown, as in many clinical investigations (Guze 1978a).

There appears to be growing recognition that diagnosis (or classification) is indispensable for clinical work and for research, in psychiatry as in the rest of medicine, primarily for effective communication, if not for thinking and planning. Questions obviously remain about the "crucial common denominators" to be used for diagnosis and how to establish the relative advantages of different choices; in other words, how to evaluate the validity of any proposed diagnostic category.

Diagnostic Validity

Eli Robins and I proposed in 1970 that the validity of any diagnostic category be based on how well it predicts etiology, pathogenesis, course, response to treatment, and associated familial psychopathology. At the same time, we recognized that for most psychiatric disorders very little is known about either etiology or pathogenesis, thus forcing us to depend mainly upon clinical course (including response to treatment), outcome, and familial illness patterns. New work in a number of fields promises that it may soon be possible to understand the pathogenesis of some conditions, but, until that is true, validation will be limited to the above variables.

Again, Kendell's view is similar: "the usefulness and validity of a classification are largely dependent on the strength of its prognostic and therapeutic implications. This suggests that boundaries should be placed in such a way that categories are as homogeneous as possible with respect to prognosis, or as a statistician would put it, so that the ratio of 'between group' to 'within group' variance is maximal in this respect" (Kendell 1975).

In this context the perspective of a leading taxonomist on certain general principles concerning classification may be helpful (Sokal 1974). R.R. Sokal points out that "all classifications aim to achieve economy of memory. The world is full of single cases: single individuals of animal or plant species, single case histories of disease, single books, rocks, or industrial concerns. By grouping numerous individual objects into a taxon, the description of the taxon subsumes the individual descriptions of the objects contained within it." (A taxon is a "set of objects . . . recognized as a group in a classificatory system.")

Sokal emphasizes the difference between "monothetic" and "polythetic" classifications. Monothetic classifications are "those in which the classes established differ by at least one property which is uniform among the members of each class." In polythetic classifications, by contrast, "taxa are groups of individuals or objects that share a large proportion of their properties but do not necessarily agree in any one property."

Sokal goes on to say that the "adoption of polythetic principles of classification negates the concept of an essence or type of any taxon. No single uniform property is required for the definition of a given group nor will any combination of characteristics necessarily define it. Thus it is extremely difficult to define class attributes for such taxa as cows or chairs. Although cows can be described as animals with four legs that give milk, a cow that only has three legs and does not give milk will still be recognized as a cow. Conversely there are other animals with four legs that give milk that are not cows. It is similarly difficult to define necessary properties for the class 'chairs.' Properties that might commonly be found in each chair might be missing in any given piece of furniture that would be recognized as a chair."

Polythetic classifications are thus based on the use of many properties or features. The diagnostic classification used in medicine is generally polythetic. Disorders with a single pathognomonic characteristic that reveals their identitiy are extremely rare in medicine and even rarer in psychiatry.

This may change for psychiatry as a result of new research findings, especially in neurobiology and genetics. Demonstrating the presence of specific brain lesions or specific genes may permit a monothetic classification for some disorders. This will require that the lesion show extremely high specificity for the particular condition or that the mode of inheritance involve complete penetrance, so that the gene is always associated with the disorder. For the great majority of clinical conditions, polythetic diagnostic criteria will continue to be necessary.

Diagnosis and Research

Because it is so important, the central place of diagnosis in medical research deserves reemphasis (Guze and Helzer 1985). Research involving clinical conditions, guided by the medical model, is concerned with the common denominators associated specifically with a given illness. The cases of such illnesses must be as homogeneous as possible, whether one is investigating cause, anatomical or chemical changes, response to treatment, or epidemiology. It is doubtful, in fact, that successful studies of cause, disease mechanisms, or treatment can be carried out if the investigator does not separate the patients into valid and maximally homogeneous diagnostic categories, consistent with knowledge at the time.

As noted above, validating a diagnosis may be divided into five phases: clinical description, laboratory studies, separation from other disorders, follow-up studies (including response to treatment), and family studies (Robins and Guze 1970). We may begin on the basis of traditional teaching, intuition, or any special experience or observation. We need as clear and unambiguous a description as possible of the defining characteristics of the index disorder, including specific criteria for inclusion or exclusion of individual patients. These defining features should encompass, whenever possible, information derived from laboratory studies of various kinds. These can include the findings from anatomical, chemical, physiological, and radiological or other imaging techniques applied to various cells, fluids, tissues, and organs. Information from psychological tests may be included as well.

Until very recently, laboratory tests have played only a limited role in this process in psychiatry because our understanding of possible pathophysiologic mechanisms has been limited. In the last few years, the situation has been changing. We are beginning to see studies utilizing a variety of laboratory indicators of different brain functions. While the results thus far are still modest and inconsistent, there is reason to be optimistic that, before too long, laboratory findings may begin to play a role in clinical psychiatry similar to their role in the rest of medicine, where they have assumed ever more important roles in diagnosis, often providing the critical information for classifying patients.

In general medicine, with the tremendous explosion of laboratory methods, classification is increasingly based primarily upon laboratory findings. And within such laboratory-defined diagnostic groups, subclassifications based upon clinical and epidemiological characteristics are possible and increasingly used (Feinstein et al. 1969a, 1969b, 1969c, 1969d, Guze 1970b). For example, classifications based upon an analysis of symptoms, signs, clinical history, and certain epidemiologic characteristics have permitted subgroupings of patients with many different disorders (including various cancers and cardiovascular disease) into categories having different prognoses and showing different responses to treatment (Guze 1970b).

This may be starting in psychiatry. Some patients with depression show resistance to dexamethasone-induced suppression of cortisol secre-

tion. Some show a decreased latency in the onset of rapid eye movement (REM) sleep. Some patients with schizophrenia have enlarged
cerebral ventricles or smaller cerebellar vermises as revealed by CAT
scans or MRIs. While such findings are also encountered in patients
with other psychiatric conditions, they still may represent alterations in
anatomy or physiology that are relevant with regard to etiology, pathogenesis, or response to treatment. Thus, these laboratory variables may
be used to help classify patients for appropriate studies.

For example, will comparisons between depressed patients who are
otherwise alike but who differ with regard to their response to dexame-
thasone or with regard to their REM latency show different responses
to different treatments? Will they show different patterns of familial illness aggregations? Some studies designed to answer such questions have
been started, but it is too early to know how well presently recognized
differences in laboratory findings will contribute to validating and
strengthening diagnostic categories.

At this point, therefore, psychiatric diagnoses are still based mainly
on the careful description and analysis of the patient's history and mental status. Some individuals begin showing psychopathology in childhood, others in early adulthood, still others only in old age. Some experience only brief, limited episodes of illness; others suffer from chronic
difficulty. Some illnesses cause little impairment; others are associated
with severe disability. Some conditions are more common in women;
others in men. Some patients never experience delusions and hallucinations; others are overwhelmed by such experiences. The same can be
said of phobias, obsessions, memory failures, mania, and learning difficulties. Many of these differences are likely to be important clues to
etiology and pathogenesis (Guze and Helzer 1985).

Ideally, the validity of any diagnostic group will depend on showing
for all of the cases within it a common etiology, a common pathogenesis, a common course and outcome, and a uniform response to intervention. Such complete diagnostic validity is unrealistic in psychiatry as
well as in medicine. In its absence, at least partial validity for psychiatric diagnoses can be inferred from a common clinical course and, in
some disorders, an increased prevalence of the same illness in the close
relatives of index cases.

Regarding the use of familial aggregation of illnesses to validate diagnosis, I have written elsewhere that "most psychiatric illnesses have

been shown to run in families, whether the investigations were designed to study hereditary or environmental causes. Independent of the question of etiology, therefore, the finding of an increased prevalence of the same disorder among the close relatives of the original patients strongly indicates that one is dealing with a valid entity" (Robins and Guze 1970). Similar hereditary and environmental factors will be operating within a family, regardless of the nature of the illness, so that it is to be expected that other members of a family will suffer from the same illness. It perhaps needs no emphasis, but most diseases tend to have familial patterns, though certainly to varying degrees.

To restate the fundamental implication of the medical model: everything—taking care of the patient, doing research, sharing experiences, thinking, and teaching—depends upon the careful examination and description of the patient's condition, in other words, on diagnosis (Goodwin and Guze 1989).

Diagnosis and Altered Physiology

Illness represents the manifestations of disturbed function within a part of the body. Each body part has only a restricted repertoire of such manifestations. In general, the same restricted repertoire will be manifested in most illnesses affecting a certain part of the body, independent of etiology, though there may be variation in the manifestations as a function of the severity and type of disturbance. In fact, the regualarity of the correlation between the manifestations of different illnesses and the pathophysiologic findings has played a central role in elucidating the normal function of the many parts of the body.

For example, as medical knowledge expanded, diagnosis and differential diagnosis increasingly reflected the recognition that edema often represented a disturbance of the heart. In time, it became clear that this edema resulted from impairment in the pumping action of the heart coupled to changes in blood flow through the kidney leading to retention of fluid in the body. Further research established the roles of various hormones in the pathophysiology of such edema. Other research led to the recognition that similar edema might result from abnormalities in the kidney itself or in the liver, and that the specific pathophysiologic processes in such cases, while overlapping somewhat with those resulting from intrinsic heart disease, showed characteristic differences as well. Through such studies, the specific roles of the heart, kidney and liver in the normal physiology involved in circulating the blood, maintaining fluid balance, and clearing the blood of certain by-products of cellular metabolism were clarified. It became clear that the heart's pumping action can be impaired through several different mechanisms: high blood pressure, coronary artery disease, valvular heart damage, and so on.

Furthermore, we saw that the heart's normal function required not only an intact pumping mechanism, but also an intact mechanism for regulating the heart rate, which depended upon a normally functioning structure called the cardiac conduction system that can likewise be deranged by a variety of different causes: endocrine disturbances (thyroid hyperactivity), coronary atherosclerosis, or valvular deformities.

We are gradually learning similar things about the brain and its parts. Our knowledge here is more rudimentary, but the same principles appear to be operating. For example, clinicians and neuroscientists now recognize surprisingly consistent correlations between certain psychotic clinical manifestations (especially hallucinations and delusions) and manipulations of the brain's dopamine system. These observations certainly suggest strongly that the dopamine system plays a significant role in certain mental functions.

At the same time, certain manifestations of illness are so ubiquitous that they probably represent derangements in one or more specific organ systems that are affected in many different conditions or suggest that in many organ systems, when they are deranged in special ways, certain cellular processes are initiated that are similar, regardless of the nature of the derangement. Fever is one example of a manifestation of illness that is present in many different conditions involving many different organs and suborgans.

The pathogenesis of fever involves the altered function of certain hypothalamic nuclei that are triggered by exogenous and endogenous molecules, often referred to as pyrogens. These molecules may be derived from pathogenic microorganisms or may be released by specific cells in the body in response to a variety of stimuli, including infections or other cell damage (Andreoli et al. 1986, Wyngaarden and Smith 1988). Another example of a widespread manifestation of illness is fatigue. Very little is known yet about its pathogenesis, but it may turn out to be analogous to fever in that here too we may be dealing with specific brain systems affected by a variety of inputs mobilized in different illnesses.

The syndrome of depression offers another example. Depression may occur alone; that is, it may be the only manifestation of the individual's illness, sometimes as a single episode, sometimes as a recurrent condition. In other cases, depression and mania may occur in the same person in a variety of sequences. In still other circumstances, depression may occur in individuals who have other pre-existing disorders, sometimes psychiatric (such as obsessional disorder, alcoholism, or schizophrenia) and sometimes general medical (such as cancer, stroke, or arthritis). It is possible that the mechanisms underlying the depressions in each of these circumstances are basically the same or at least share certain features. When the pathophysiology of depression is better understood, we are likely to know much more about the structures and functions of the relevant brain systems in experiencing normal moods.

If general medical experience is a good guide, the clarification of these questions concerning psychiatric illnesses will require a great deal of research in which there will be repeated interaction between clinical studies of the disorders and animal studies designed to learn more about the brain's anatomy and physiology. In the rest of medicine, diagnosis based primarily on symptoms and signs has proven to be useful only up to a point; further advances depended upon new technologies and advances in basic science. The same sequence of development is likely to be necessary in psychiatry.

Some Insights from Neurology

This same set of issues has been addressed by neurologists studying the anatomical correlates of various neuropsychological abnormalities (Damasio and Damasio 1989). In discussing their own work, the Damasios note that a "pertinent methodological issue relates to the neuropsychological taxonomies. Although none of our current research is based on any syndromatic classification of the classical neuropsychological disorders, clearly, communication among clinicians and researchers must rely, for the foreseeable future, on the use of numerous convenient syndrome and symptom designations. However, whenever we use those terms, it should not be taken to mean that we subscribe necessarily, to either the full classificatory validity of those entities, or to the neuropsychological or neurophysiological accounts that have been traditionally attached to them."

They then go on to explain their position. "As in the case with any taxonomic entity in medicine, clinical syndromes are characterized by a cluster of co-occurring signs that signifies the presence of a given disease process. In each instance of classification, the cluster may be surrounded by a varied degree of additional signs or by none at all. There need not be any causal relation among the signs, mere coincidence being sufficient. A syndrome's clinical validity is measurable by the accuracy of the predictions it generates."

They follow up with an important point that probably applies to all classifications in the broad field of medicine and not just to their own field of specialization. "In neurology, and especially in the neurology of cognition, the syndrome is used to predict a lesion location rather than a disease process, and its validity is thus checked in relation to an anatomical prediction, rather than a prediction of pathological process. This poses problems because numerous forms of pathology can affect the same location, with different consequences. Another problem derives from the design and workings of the nervous system in relation to cognition: the distributiveness and relative redundancy of functions within and across anatomical networks is such that similar, albeit not precisely equal, syndromes can result from dysfunction in different neural sites. Consequently, when factors such as individual biological and educational variables are added, the accuracy of syndrome-based predictions can be reduced. We believe that, provided expert judgement is exercised, syndromes remain extremely useful tools for clinicians."

These authors have encapsulated the issues concerning clinical diagnosis very well. It seems to me that their ideas apply equally well to psychiatric disorders but, as yet, we still have too little anatomical knowledge to add to the clinical syndrome so as to improve diagnosis overall. Many psychiatrists believe that this situation is beginning to change. It may not be very long before we will be able to depend upon consistent correlations between some specific clinical syndromes and the neuroanatomical distribution of abnormal brain processes.

Diagnosis and the Roles of Temperament and Socioeconomic Factors

Arguing for the central role of diagnosis in psychiatry or general medicine is fully compatible with recognizing the roles of temperament, social and economic background, and family interactions in the development and course of illness. The medical model can easily accommodate the possibility that an individual's personality and social and psychological environments may prove of great importance in illness, but their role cannot be assessed correctly if diagnosis is ignored. Furthermore, while differences in temperament, social and economic backgrounds, and family interactions may play important roles, it is unlikely that such differences will prove to be as important as the nature, and hence the diagnosis, of the illness itself. In other words, the information conveyed by a valid diagnosis predicts what will happen to the patient's health status better than anything else, including the patient's personality, psychosocial environment, and economic condition.

If one set of social or psychologic factors plays a role in the development of cancer of the lung and another set in cancer of the cervix, a study that combines patients with both types of cancer will most likely fail to recognize the differential importance of psychosocial factors. To illustrate: there is considerable evidence relating prior sexual history to cancer of the cervix, but not to most other cancers (except for the characteristic cancers that complicate AIDS). Thus, studying the role of past sexual experience in cancer patients generally is not likely to uncover the association with cervical cancer. Similarly, if certain sociocultural factors are important in schizophrenia but not in depression, this is not likely to be discovered in studies that ignore the importance of the diagnostic distinction.

The medical model, instead of denying the importance of psychosocial factors in illness and health, can contribute importantly to demonstrating and testing the significance of such factors. It is interesting to note, for example, that certain birth difficulties have been reported to be more prominent in schizophrenics without schizophrenia in their close relatives than in those with such relatives (Gottesman and Shields 1982), indicating that it may be important to separate patients by family illness patterns as well as by diagnosis in studies of the possible effects of early life experiences on the development of schizophrenia.

Diagnosis and Comorbidity

Comorbidity is a relatively new concept in psychiatry that bears directly upon psychiatric diagnosis. It refers to the presence of multiple clinical syndromes in the same patient. The concept derived from the relatively new field of clinical epidemiology (Feinstein 1985).

Clinical epidemiology corresponds closely to what I have been referring to as clinical research, the intersection between traditional epidemiological and laboratory approaches to medical research, using concepts and techniques from both fields. Comorbid conditions are important in clinical research because they can play a role in the ascertainment of cases, compliance, response to treatment, and outcome.

For example, a comorbid condition might lead the patient to seek help sooner and, therefore, result in the patient's index condition being recognized and treated earlier than if no other disorder were present, possibly improving the outcome. On the other hand, the comorbid condition's treatment might adversely affect the patient's response to treatment for the index illness, leading to more severe side effects and noncompliance. Furthermore, medication for one of the disorders might alter the metabolism of the drug directed against the other disorder, influencing blood levels of the drugs and in turn the clinical response. In other circumstances, a comorbid condition might reduce the patient's longevity, thus affecting the apparent prognosis of the other illness. Or, a comorbid condition might influence the decision to use certain treatments for the other disorder because the combined treatments seem too risky. In all these ways, comorbidity can be, and often turns out to be, an important issue in many clinical studies as well as in clinical practice.

Comorbidity is a very difficult concept to work with unless diagnostic criteria are relatively clear and unambiguous for each of the comorbid conditions. This important point is particularly relevant to psychiatry where diagnostic validity is not yet as firm as it is in other areas of medicine.

In psychiatry, the concept of comorbidity has not been consistently applied with all of this in mind. Instead, it has been used to refer to the coexistence of more than one clinical syndrome in a given patient, such as the presence of panic or phobic symptoms with depression or substance abuse with antisocial personality. We do not know yet whether depression associated with panic or phobic symptoms is validly different from depression without such additional symptoms, though relevant data are becoming available (Guze 1990, Maser and Cloninger 1990). Based upon our current ideas concerning validity, we need well-controlled studies of clinical course, response to treatment, outcome, and familial illness aggregation before we can know the best way to classify the different groups of patients suffering from comorbid conditions.

A major reason for the recent and growing interest in psychiatric comorbidity is to be found in the trend seen in DSM-III-R and in the development of DSM-IV to eliminate diagnostic hierarchies and rules to exclude diagnoses under certain circumstances (Frances 1990). For example, in the past, an intercurrent depression in a particular patient with schizophrenia would not result in a second diagnosis of depression. Now the diagnostician is forced to use multiple diagnoses because current rules make few allowances for the possibility that one syndrome, depression, for example, might be only part of an underlying and preexisting condition (e.g., schizophrenia). Previously, such patients would receive only one diagnosis, schizophrenia; now the same patient will receive two diagnoses: depression and schizophrenia.

One approach to this important issue, again borrowing from general medicine, is to differentiate between "primary" and "secondary" syndromes (Feighner et al. 1972, Guze 1990, Guze et al. 1971, Woodruff et al. 1967). This was first proposed for depression, but it can also be applied to anxiety and other syndromes. Primary depressions were defined as those that arise in an individual without a history of any psychiatric disorder except for previous episodes of depression or mania. Secondary depressions were divided into two groups. The first included depressions that develop in individuals with a preexisting nonaffective psychiatric disorder, which may or may not still be present. The second included depressions that develop in individuals suffering from life-threatening or incapacitating medical illnesses and that parallel the course of the illnesses (Feighner et al. 1972, Guze et al. 1971, Robins and Guze 1972).

A number of controlled studies have evaluated the validity of this distinction. The results have shown that secondary depressions in patients with preexisting anxiety disorders (panic disorder and generalized anxiety disorder), schizophrenia, alcoholism, and hysteria (Briquet's syndrome) are not associated with an increased frequency of primary depressive illnesses in first-degree relatives (Cloninger et al. 1981, Guze 1990, Guze et al. 1983, 1986). Of equal interest is the finding that in these same disorders, secondary depression was also not familial; that is, the first-degree relatives of index patients with secondary depressions were not more likely to experience secondary depressions than were the relatives of index patients without secondary depression, when the index patients were matched for primary diagnosis.

One report (Pearlson 1990), on the other hand, suggests that at least some secondary depressions seen in patients suffering from Alzheimer's disease may be familial. First-degree relatives of patients with Alzheimer's disease and secondary depression reported more primary depressions than did relatives of patients with Alzheimer's disease who did not have secondary depressions.

Much more needs to be done before psychiatry can hope to utilize effectively the concept of comorbidity. In dealing with psychiatric conditions, it is important to recognize the relative uncertainty and ambiguity about the limits of many of our diagnostic categories. It is not clear on any *a priori* grounds, for example, whether intercurrent anxiety symptoms during an episode of prolonged depression should be viewed as part of the depressive illness or as a distinct disorder. Similar questions arise when an episode of depression develops in an individual with a long history of recurrent anxiety symptoms and panic attacks.

The primary and secondary distinction, based largely on temporal sequencing, offers one practical strategy for beginning to study the issues. This strategy is not without important, unresolved questions, however. It is not yet clear what ought to be the proper approach to deciding on the time of onset of the secondary disorder. For example, is the second disorder dated from the time it meets the full diagnostic criteria or from the onset of its first symptom? Similarly, what if the complete diagnostic criteria for the first disorder are not fulfilled until after the initial symptom of the second disorder is present?

For such reasons as well as our continuing ignorance abut the pathogenesis of most psychiatric conditions, psychiatric comorbidity is more problematic than is the case in areas of medicine in which the discrimination between disorders is on a firmer basis. Furthermore, comorbidity presents different problems depending upon whether we are considering two psychiatric conditions or one psychiatric disorder and a general medical one. In the latter circumstances, the diagnostic boundary of the medical disorder is usually less ambiguous, making it easier to establish the presence of comorbidity. If the medical disorder is not clearly defined and delineated from other illnesses, comorbidity can prove as difficult as when the illnesses are all psychiatric.

Comorbidity depends upon clear diagnostic criteria, reasonable in-dependent evidence concerning the validity of each diagnosis, and some attention to the chronology of the separate conditions. Comorbidity ought to be considered a form of diagnostic classification. As such, comorbid combinations need validation in the same way that all diagnostic cate-gories are validated. We need answers to questions such as the follow-ing. What are the epidemiological characteristics, course and outcome, response to intervention, and familial illness patterns of specific co-morbid combinations? Does the study of various comorbid combina-tions contribute to our understanding of the etiology or pathogenesis of the individual conditions in a comorbid grouping (Guze 1990)?

Some Concluding Remarks

Diagnostic practice inevitably reflects the evolving state of knoweldge concerning all aspects of illness, from etiology and pathogenesis to epi-demiology and response to intervention. Diagnosis is merely a short-hand way of incorporating knowledge concerning all these matters. Not rarely, however, whether in clinical practice or in research, diagnosti-cians act as though the knowledge base for the diagnostic categories is much stronger and more complete than it really is. In my own expe-rience, clinical and investigative, confident diagnoses cannot be made in a substantial minority of patients. In some of my studies, as many as a third of the cases remain undiagnosed. This results from a number of circumstances: the diagnostic criteria are not fully met but no other diagnosis seems reasonable, more than one disorder seems to be present but the temporal sequence is not definite, highly atypical features are present that shake my confidence in the apparent diagnosis, and so on.

Failure to recognize and understand present limitations in our diag-nostic abilities, coupled with the undesirable consequence of forcing patients into categories that are not truly appropriate, can only under-mine the usefulness of diagnosis. Cases should be assigned to categories only when they truly meet the diagnostic criteria. Otherwise, the cate-gories will be diluted by the atypical or uncertain cases. This inevitably leads to reduced validity. Validity is the gold standard for judging any diagnostic category and comparing different diagnostic approaches. Esthetic and political considerations and *a priori* assumptions must give way to it (Guze 1989b).

"Undiagnosed" need not be the equivalent of unknown. Undiagnosed cases can be divided into subgroups based upon the diagnostic problems. Examples might include "undiagnosed: schizophrenia vs. psychotic depression" or "undiagnosed: ?depression, too few or inconsistent features." Such characterization of the illnesses can identify the diagnostic problem and increase the likelihood of ultimately clarifying it.

Reading psychiatric reports in which the recognition of undiagnosed cases is not evident makes me wonder how much confidence to place on the author's findings. Diagnosis is not an end in itself, but rather an essential process to increase our understanding of illness and its treatment. As such, it requires very high standards in its application.

To repeat, diagnostic categories and criteria will change as we learn more. Traditional criteria will be modified or replaced by new criteria. New parameters will become important: neuroimaging, biochemical or physiological processes, personality features, social factors, and so on. Clinical symptoms and signs will take on special significance depending upon the presence or absence of a particular laboratory finding or epidemiological characteristic (Guze 1989b). Only failure to treat diagnosis seriously will slow the pace of advance.

A remaining issue concerning diagnosis must be addressed, namely, the differential value of the categorical approach compared to the dimensional one. The categorical approach is obviously derived from traditional medical practice, where entities such as gout, diabetes, or cholera are used. The dimensional approach, in which individuals are assigned to a rank in some distribution curve, is widely used in psychology where psychological testing tends to have a quantitative perspective. In actual practice, both styles of diagnosis are used in both professions. The choice generally reflects one's assumption concerning the nature of the fundamental process underlying the clinical condition.

If one assumes that the disorder is based upon some qualitative deviation, a categorical classification is logical, though it can be and often is coupled with an additional dimensional subclassification reflecting degrees of severity. On the other hand, if one assumes that the basis for the disorder is a trait that is widely distributed in the population and that overt illness is a matter of being at the end of a distribution curve, one prefers a dimensional scale for classification.

Clinical medicine, including psychiatry, uses both forms of classification. It has already been noted, in Chapter 1, that hypertension may be regarded as a qualitative deviation, as in certain forms of renal disease, while in other cases, where the cause is unclear, it may simply be regarded as a higher than normal level of blood pressure, which is normally distributed in the population.

Personality disorders may also be viewed from both the categorical and quantiative perspectives. A personality disorder may simply be an individual at one or the other end of a normal population distribution. Another person's behavior may have been profoundly affected by a specific metabolic disturbance, such as vitamin B-12 deficiency or the chronic use of a drug like amphetamine.

Often it is not clear which perspective is more fully justified to interpret the available data. Based on a number of family studies, for example, there appears to be an association within families between schizophrenia and schizotypal personality disorder. Some are inclined to view schizotypal personality as a mild manifestation of schizophrenia. They believe that it is possible to see all gradations from mild schizotypal personality to severe schizophrenia. Others prefer to view schizotypal personality as an important predisposing factor for the development of schizophrenia, which they see as requiring an additional etiological factor—perhaps a psychosocial experience or brain damage—to produce the full disorder. The problem is highlighted by patients who develop schizophrenia without evidence of a preexisting schizotypal personality.

In the final analysis, the differences between the two perspectives may not be very important. It is now appreciated that some traits that appear to vary in the population along a normal distribution curve result from the interaction of a small number of discrete genes, as few as three to five. Thus, we must bear in mind that even phenotypes with these characteristic quantitative population distributions may result from the combined impact of *qualitatively* discrete genes.

The vital place of diagnosis in psychiatry is at the core of the medical model. As already emphasized, diagnosis at any point in time is simply a shorthand way of summarizing knowledge about a particular clinical disorder. The validity of any specific diagnosis must be based upon the extent and depth of our knowledge concerning the clinical picture, clinical course, response to treatment, etiology, and pathogenesis. The more we learn about these, the greater our confidence in the diagnostic criteria. Thus, research is the key to improved diagnosis.

4

Biology and Psychiatry

Defining Biological Psychiatry

Biological psychiatry, like the medical model it is so inextricably en-
twined with, is more than an assumption about etiology and pathogenesis. It represents a perspective for conceptualizing psychiatric disorders
in such a way as to integrate psychiatry more closely into the biological
sciences. It is not synonymous with prescribing medication, though it
has no difficulty accepting the use of appropriate medications. It places
the brain and its structure and functions in health and illness at the
center of interest and study.

Biological psychiatry is perhaps the inevitable outcome of following
the medical model. It is the attempt to imbed the medical model within
the matrix of our knowledge about evolution, neurobiology, cognitive
science, and genetics because this offers the most comprehensive and
inclusive framework for dealing with psychiatric illness (Guze 1989a).
It links the medical model to the major issues and concerns of the
philosophy of science by taking seriously philosophy's continuing de-
bates about mind-brain relationships, consciousness, language, knowing, epistemology, free will, determinism, and so forth, all of which are
of interest to modern biology as well (see Chapter 6).

Biology provides not only a tremendous amount of information at
many different levels of complexity, but it also offers strategic concepts
that have evolved from the scientific study of living creatures over many
generations. Among these are the importance of individual variation
within nearly all categories of biological phenomena, of recognizing
that living creatures may utilize many different ways of carrying out
what appear to be similar functions, of adaptation for understanding the
evolution of the species and the development of the individual, and of
what have been called "programs" as "teleonomic" alternatives to "te-

leological" explanations for the behavior of individual creatures (Mayr 1982, 1988, Young 1978, 1987). (This will be further discussed below.)

Such concepts and their associated research strategies are basic to the description of biological psychiatry proposed here, a description that acknowledges our present ignorance and incomplete understanding, but offers a framework for trying to reduce that ignorance and, at the same time, for thinking about and trying to help our patients. Biological psychiatry, when conceived so that these concepts from modern biology are central, is necessarily interested in the origin, development, structure, and function of brain systems that subserve adaptation and explain individual variation in such adaptation, especially with regard to the teleonomic programs that Mayr (Mayr 1988, page 49) defines as "coded or prearranged information that controls a process (or behavior) leading it toward a given end." Mayr emphasizes that a program is something "material" and that it exists prior to the initation of the teleonomic process. In other words, such programs are based upon cellular and molecular systems that have evolved to guide the organism's responses to various stimuli.

Implications of Biological Psychiatry

The origins, evolution, development, structure, and function of such adaptive systems are being studied at different levels: that of species and other groups, that of the individual organism, that of bodily organs, and that of isolated cells and molecules. Regardless of the level of investigation, modern biologists recognize that all forms of life have adapted to their environments through the processes of evolution and that they are continuing to adapt in many ways to a wide range of environmental conditions. For them, the primary focus always includes the adapting organism, its capacities, limitations, and variations.

Medicine may be viewed as a form of applied biology, in which health and illness are recognized as manifestations of the organism's adaptation over time to its changing environment. Biological psychiatry comprises a set of ideas and assumptions that lead to the same way of thinking about psychiatric disorders. Like the rest of medicine, biological psy-

chiatry is based on the belief that increased knowledge about the anatomy and physiology of the body, in this case especially the brain, is
vital for improved practice. But it is not so much based on current
knowledge of anatomy and physiology in psychiatric conditions as on a
strategic way of thinking and the expectation that this will lead to the
relevant knowledge.

A similar view was set forth cogently in 1983 by Charles Scriver, a
Canadian geneticist, in his Rutherford Lecture (Scriver 1984). "It is said
that genes propose and experiences dispose. Biological adaptation (to fit
with the experiences of life) implies functional and structural homeostasis. Disadaptation (the undoing of fitness, that is, morbidity, disease)
occurs when experience overwhelms homeostasis or phenotypic variation undermines it. Human disease has social and cultural contexts, but
is also measurable in the biological dimensions of viability, development, reproduction, and longevity. Heritability is a description of 'cause'
and, for some classes of disease, heritability is high in modern society
relative to the past."

Evolution is the bedrock of biology as we know it today (Mayr 1982).
Scriver (1984) extended this point to medicine: "An evolutionary view
of human health and disease is not surprising or new; it is merely inevitable in the face of evidence and time."

From the perspective of psychiatry, the central fact is that evolution
has shaped the development of the brain, which is the organ of mental
functions. The process of evolution has involved selection: choosing
from existing, varied possibilities and combinations (Margolis 1988). Such
choices have ultimtely led to modified and new forms and functions.
All brain structures and functions, including those involved in mental
activities, such as perception, learning, thought, memory, emotions,
and communication, represent the results of evolution. All mental capacities, including the ability to feel, be aware, recognize, remember,
learn, talk, think, depend upon the "programs" of the evolved brain.
This wonderfully evolved brain, with its remarkable complexity, makes
possible our rich mental and emotional capacities. It also makes possible our many forms of psychopathology. *The very complexity of the
brain provides many places where subtle but important variations in
structure or function can develop.*

Biology has been transformed by modern genetics, especially molecular genetics. It is estimated that the human genome contains approxi-

mately three billion nucleotide pairs and that a substantial share are devoted to programming the brain (Siegel et al. 1989). The sequencing and arrangements of these nucleotides determine the repertoire of our sensitivity and our responses to all sorts of stimuli.

The growth and development of the brain depend on the DNA sequences of the genotype. These sequence patterns provide the potential for the epigenetic processes (genotype-environment interactions) that lead to the remarkable variations seen among individuals and to the powerful effects of cultural evolution. The brain-coding genes make possible language, memory, and abstract thinking that, in turn, facilitate the development of art, music, science, religion, philosophy, politics, and all the other manifestations of human culture. Here again, the size and complexity of the genotye offer many opportunities for certain phenotypes, interacting with certain environments, to be expressed in one or another form of psychopathology.

Genotype-environment interaction is probably not a simple matter. For instance, many interpret the absence of complete concordance in the study of twins with various psychiatric disorders as indicating the role of environmental factors in the etiology of the disorders, C. D. Mellon and L. D. Clark (1990) argue that "decreased concordance is certainly not proof that nongenetic forms of major psychiatric illness exist." Instead they insist that "somatic genome alterations, developmental plasticity in the form of nonprogrammed random developmental events, and . . . phenotypic plasticity using the model of chaos theory" may account for the absence of complete concordance. The research cited by these authors deals with the production of antibodies, the etiology of certain cancers, chromosomal mosaicism, mobile genetic elements, and extrachromosomal DNA, none of which has yet proven relevant to common psychiatric disorders. Their thesis is only that failure to find complete concordance need not always mean that a significant environmental etiological factor is operating. Furthermore, it is certainly important to keep in mind that the environment in genotype-environment interaction includes many factors that are not part of the psychosocially significant environment commonly considered to be etiologically related to psychiatric conditions. Ingested chemicals, infectious agents, foodstuffs of all kinds, and climatic variables are among the other possibly relevant environmental factors to be considered.

What to Expect from Neuroscience

Returning to the growth and development of the brain, the neurosciences are evolving rapidly, but knowledge about brain processes underlying higher mental functions is still rudimentary. Much has been learned
about the way individual cells work and interact, but understanding
about coordination and integration of large assemblies of cells during
mental events is only beginning (Changeaux 1985, Edelman 1987,
Edelman and Mountcastle 1978, Kandel and Schwartz 1985, Posner
1989, Young 1987), and experimental approaches are underway (Posner
et al. 1988, Sawaguchi and Goldman-Rakic 1991).

We still know very little about the storage and coding of memories
and language and about how abstract ideas are developed. But those of
us who accept the central place of biology in mental functioning are
confident that the brain is involved in all of this. Furthermore, it seems
highly plausible that the great variability in brain development and
function, recognized in experimental animals as well as in humans,
offers a basis for ultimately explaining at least some of the variation seen
in humans with regard to temperament, emotionality, and other parameters of adjustment. Finally, biology provides a central place, through
epigenesis, for environmental forces that might influence learning, personality, perception, sexuality, and many other important features of
human life. Ethology and ecology are two important disciplines within
biology that have long recognized explicitly that all forms of life are
shaped by and in turn shape their environments. These fields have
demonstrated clearly the inseparable linkages between organisms and
their environments.

Within medicine epidemiology has long reflected the same fundamental understanding. We know that all sorts of important factors can
profoundly influence growth and development, behavior, and, of course,
health and illness. These factors include geography, climate, social and
economic conditions, amount and variety of food, exposure to a wide
range of polluting substances, educational experiences, family constel-
lations and arrangements, and much more. Much is unknown about
how these factors operate at the physiological level, but beginnings have
been made in a number of areas (Changeaux 1985, Purves and Lichtman 1985).

To summarize the argument thus far, a broad approach to biology and thus to biological psychiatry includes the fundamental premise that all forms of life, including humans in health and disease, are best conceptualized within an adaptive network of evolution, homeostasis, and individual variation. Biology is more than anatomy and physiology, but, at the same time, these disciplines are indispensable for a comprehensive understanding. Biology requires these three perspectives (evolution, homeostasis, individual variation) to understand structure and function under different conditions and circumstances.

Some psychiatrists will ask in what way biological psychiatry, as described here, differs from what they call the biopsychosocial model. This latter model, like biological psychiatry, explicitly recognizes the broad spectrum of factors relevant to psychiatric disorders. It provides a place for evolution, neurobiology, genetics, subjective psychological experiences, and sociocultural contexts. It differs, however, by not placing the brain and those of its processes that subserve mental phenomena at the hub of psychiatric thinking. All of medicine can be viewed from a biopsychosocial perspective, but *in the rest of medicine, the body and its processes are recognized implicitly as the hub of medical thinking*. The medical model, inseparably linked to biological psychiatry, specifies the same approach to psychiatric conditions. In the end, that is the key difference between the two approaches: the biopsychosocial model specifies no hierarchy or priority among its various elements; the medical model underlying biological psychiatry specifies a hierarchy among its elements for conceptualizing and practicing psychiatry.

Psychopathology and Neuroscience

Medicine has come to appreciate the importance of individual variation—based upon genetics, development, and other experiences—in explaining the etiology and pathogenesis of disease. It is just this sort of variation in the anatomy and physiology of the brain that is at the heart of biological psychiatry. While very little is known yet about the details, biological psychiatrists assume that many forms of psychopathology are the result of different responses of the individual's brain to the circumstances of his or her life, and that these differences in response follow from differences in the way the brain has developed and functions.

If this assumption were wrong, if it turned out that *few, if any* of the conditions that psychiatry is concerned with are the result of differences in brain development, structure, or function, then biological psychiatry might not make sense. If all or most psychiatric patients developed their disorders through learning processes that are essentially independent of brain variability, an emphasis on biology could be regarded as unjustified. If most individuals exposed to a particular pattern of childrearing or other social conditioning developed a particular disorder, psychiatry might need neuroscience less than cultural anthropology and social psychology.

There is no convincing evidence, however, that most individuals exposed to any widespread, psychologically meaningful experience develop a particular psychiatric disorder. In published studies, only a minority of individuals do so. Therefore, various vulnerabilities or diatheses, usually hypothesized to be the result of various bodily variations, have been suggested to account for the findings. Sometimes, such vulnerabilities have been attributed to certain previous psychosocial experiences (Brown and Harris 1978), but results from controlled prospective studies about the contributions of psychosocial experiences to vulnerability are still inconsistent (Champion 1990, Tennant 1983, 1988, Tennant and Bebbington 1978, Tennant et al. 1980).

I am not arguing here that psychologically meaningful experiences are irrelevant to the development of psychiatric disorders. But, in the majority of instances in which such connections seem to exist, the experiences consist primarily of the kinds of troubles most people encounter during their lives, usually without becoming sick (Guze and Helzer 1985). This suggests that such experiences play less than a crucial role in the development of these disorders.

We must direct our attention to specific vulnerabilities if we are to achieve significant scientific understanding and effective therapeutic intervention. For example, while nearly everyone grieves after the death of a close relative or friend, only a minority go on to develop serious depressions and very few will commit suicide. We need studies designed to describe possible vulnerability *before* the onset of the clinical condition and then show that the specific hypothesized vulnerability, whether psychological or physiological, is significantly predictive of depression or suicide. And, since the loss of close relatives or friends is universal, identifying specific vulnerabilities is likely to prove most advantageous, scientifically and clinically.

Furthermore, intervention to reduce or eliminate the difficulties, dis-appointments, frustrations, and pressures of daily life seems extremely difficult and highly unlikely to be very successful, except perhaps in special circumstances. Psychotherapeutic efforts (see Chapter 5) may be directed toward this goal, but they are likely to be successful primarily to the degree that the patient is able to change his or her responses to life circumstances.

A Useful Example from General Medicine

Often a conceptual problem in psychiatry may be clarified by looking at similar circumstances in the rest of medicine. Coronary artery disease offers just such an example that can illuminate the issues concerning the causal role of psychologically meaningful experiences. Certain man-ifestations of coronary atherosclerosis, those that result from transient myocardial ischemia, are typically brought on by physical exertion or emotion-provoking situations. These observations have been recognized for generations, but they do not challenge the belief that coronary heart disease is best conceptualized within a broad biological framework, in which efforts to understand the genetic and epigenetic factors leading to differential vulnerability to coronary atherosclerosis offer the most promising research strategy. Furthermore, few are proposing that inter-ventions to reduce physical activity or emotion-provoking circumstances will be of major importance.

At the same time, however, the *apparently* favorable effects on rates of coronary artery disease of reduced consumption of animal fats and total calories suggest that specific environmental changes can sometimes be very helpful. The possible role of personality as a risk factor for cor-onary atherosclerosis in no way contravenes the biological view of this important condition. In fact, growing interest in possible associations between personality and various brain modulating neurotransmitter sys-tems raises the strong probability that personality is itself a most impor-tant manifestation of the epigenetic development of these neural systems (Cloninger 1986, 1987).

The same concepts widely accepted for coronary artery disease seem appropriate for conditions such as schizophrenia, mania, depression, obsessional disorders, and so on. As an example, few today continue to

put forward the notion of the schizophrenigenic mother with her al-
leged ambivalent and controlling style of dealing with her children. While
this was a very popular and widely accepted hypothesis a couple of de-
cades ago (and devastating to the already beleaguered mothers of very
sick offspring), it is now largely discredited because its supporters never
presented systematic, controlled data to support it. Even if the theory
still retained credibility, it would be necessary to ask why only a minority of children raised by these mothers developed schizophrenia and
whether all schizophrenics had such mothers.

It could also be asked whether some mothers of schizophrenic children might themselves suffer from a partial form of the disorder, thus
suggesting that the familial interaction might reflect a shared genetic
causal factor rather than a psychosocial one, or at least that both kinds
of factors might be operating.

In contrast, there is very strong evidence for some genetic predisposition to the disorder (Gottesman and Shields 1982), based on many
twin and adoption studies in several different countries showing strong
correlations in the prevalence of schizophrenia according to genetic
closeness. And evidence is steadily growing that there are a number of
apparent structural changes in the brains of schizophrenic patients, including enlarged cerebral ventricles, smaller cerebellar vermises, and
changes in regional blood flow in different areas of the brain using pos-
itron emission tomography (PET) (Goodwin and Guze 1989).

It seems highly plausible that what is called psychopathology represents, at least in part, the manifestations of disordered processes in various brain systems that mediate psychological functions within a genotype-environment interaction framework (Mayr 1982, 1988, Purves and
Lichtman 1985, Ruse 1986). There is no longer a place for the *tabula
rasa* assumption about the mind for any species, let alone for humans
(Changeaux 1985, Mayr 1982, Young 1978). We are all born with
powerful predispositions, sometimes called programs, that determine what
we repond to and how we respond.

Resistance to Biological Psychiatry

Despite arguments like these, resistance to the thesis that biology plays
a fundamental role in the development of psychiatric disorders is not

uncommon. Many believe that accepting a biological view, especially a genetic view, of psychopathology is tantamount to hopelessness about treatment or prevention. Some believe that the etiology of psychopathology is to be found primarily in social, economic, or political conditions. They may even claim that biological psychiatrists "blame the victims" instead of the system for their disorders and disabilities.

Others have religious reasons for opposing biological psychiatry. They fear that it will weaken or destroy the basis for "free will" and undermine religious faith by questioning humankind's "special place" in the universe. Still others have philosophical grounds for their resistance. They are skeptical that neuroscience will ever be able to account for "free will," consciousness, or other complex mental phenomena because the very goal of trying to explain mental content in terms of neural substrates is the worst sort of reductionism, indeed a "category error" (Charlton 1990). They argue that there is no possibility of connecting descriptions of mental content with descriptions of the brain because "they are not saying the same things in different ways but are actually about different things."

Despite these criticisms, there are strong reasons for concluding that they are either unfounded or unduly pessimistic. Medical advances have shown conclusively that many genetically or otherwise biologically conditioned disorders, such as diabetes, gout, and epilepsy, as a few examples, can be effectively treated. Furthermore, it is beyond doubt that the more we have learned about etiology and pathogenesis, the more we have been able to intervene somewhere in the process leading to pathology, illness, and death. In addition, as discussed earlier, there is nothing in modern biological theory that denies important places for culture, political systems, and economic circumstances in the development of illness. Lastly, it is hard to visualize translating observations about social and cultural arrangements predisposing to psychopathology into a hopeful strategy for intervention. Changing culture or socal systems is extremely difficult.

With regard to philosophical perspectives, there is no doubt that consciousness, free will, and all the richness of mental life are still largely beyond neuroscience. Perhaps they will always remain so. But predicting the future of scientific understanding has always been very difficult. Who, a generation back, predicted the tremendous developments in genetics? Who, today, can categorically assert that it will never be possible to identify and understand the way the brain codes and stores information? Who can even guess at the profound impact of such knowledge on our conceptual schemes of mental life?

It is a hopeful sign that modern biology and modern philosophy are reaching out to each other, trying to understand the other's questions, methods, and concerns (Changeaux 1985, Churchland 1986, Churchland and Churchland 1990, Rosenberg 1988, Young 1987). Such interaction may lead to the recognition that many philosophical concerns can be reinterpreted and redefined so as to permit greater specificity and more focused debate, perhaps on occasion resulting in answers that will be more satisfactory to both philosophers and biologists. This applies to free will, for example, which is discussed in Chapter 6 (Dennett 1984).

We are starting to recognize and appreciate that there may be evolutionary and genetic roots for at least some aspects of humankind's religious, ethical, and moral capacities (Ruse 1986). For example, it is conceivable that neural processes underlying the selfless devotion of mothers to their offspring, evident in many species, might also bear on evolutionary relationships with other behaviors considered ethical or moral. While this is certainly highly speculative, it may suggest possibilities for future research.

No psychiatrist, including those who accept the biological basis of psychiatry, can ignore the important roles of culture, socioeconomic circumstances, ethical considerations, and religion in trying to understand fully the development, course, and outcome of all sorts of psychiatric conditions. At the same time, however, these important matters must be integrated into a comprehensive biological framework. Cultural anthropology, philosophy, and sociology may all make significant contributions to the fullest understanding of psychopathology and its treatment, but only to the degree that they take into appropriate consideration human biology.

Disturbances in mental functions are at the center of psychiatric interest and concern. As a clinical science, psychiatry depends upon our understanding of the brain. On the foundation of such understanding, other disciplines, such as anthropology, sociology, philosophy, and ethics, can make their fullest contributions in helping understand psychiatric disorders. From this point of view the assertion has therefore been made that psychiatry can never be other than biological (Guze 1989a).

Risks in Biological Psychiatry and Other Models

One other very important issue has been raised in arguments against a central role for biology in psychiatric disorders. This issue may account for the reluctance of some to agree to this central role even when they are not concerned with the questions and reservations discussed above. It relates to the terrible example described vividly and convincingly by Robert J. Lifton (Lifton 1986), himself a psychiatrist, of how in Nazi Germany biological ideas were linked to a political and social ideology that countenanced and justified the murder of millions of innocent people and the sterilization of many others.

It is very sobering to realize the extent to which the vision and goals of Hitler and the Nazi movement were derived from and enthusiastically supported by many members of the German medical profession, including psychiatrists. This was the result of their overlapping beliefs about genetics in general and about eugenics in particular, leading to the conclusion that genetically conditioned illnesses were hopeless and that the state had the responsibility to weed out those unfit to live and procreate. Lifton has marshalled convincing evidence for his conclusion that the "Nazification of the medical profession—a key aspect of the transition from sterilization to direct medical killing—was achieved by a combination of ideological enthusiasm and systematic terror."

No psychiatrist interested in the relationship between biology and psychiatry can fail to be disturbed on learning that Dr. Ernst Rüdin (Lifton 1986, pages 27–29), a pioneer in the study of the genetics of psychiatric illness, was also the "predominant medical presence in the Nazi sterilization program. . . . Rüdin became a close associate of Alfred Ploetz in establishing the German Society for Racial Hygiene. Rüdin was an indefatigable researcher and saw as his mission the application of Mendelian laws and eugenic principles to psychiatry."

Dr. Ernst Rüdin joined the Nazi party "in 1937 at the age of sixty. From his prestigious position as director of the Research Institute for Psychiatry of the Kaiser William Society in Munich, he worked closely with a regime whose commitment to genetic principles he applauded, and was one of the principal architects of the sterilization laws." Further, "in a special issue of his journal . . . [*Archive of Racial and*

Social Biology], celebrating ten years of National Socialist rule, Rüdin extolled Hitler and the movement for its 'decisive . . . path-breaking step toward making racial hygiene a fact among the German people . . . and inhibiting the propagation of the congenitally ill and inferior.' He praised both the Nuremberg Laws for 'preventing the further penetration of the German gene pool by Jewish blood,' and the SS for 'its ultimate goal, the creation of a special group of medically superior and healthy people of the German Nordic type.' "

Lifton makes the very significant point that "while a few doctors resisted, and large numbers had little sympathy for the Nazis, *as a profession* German physicians offered themselves to the regime. So did most other professions; but with doctors, that gift included using their intellectual authority to justify and carry out medicalized killing."

In placing their professional authority at the service of Nazism, physicians were joined by others including Konrad Lorenz, who was awarded a Nobel Prize many years later for his work on ethology. His position is quoted by Lifton (Lifton 1986, page 134) from the *Journal of Applied Psychology* and the *Science of Character*, volume 59, 1940: "It must be the duty of racial hygiene to be attentive to a more severe elimination of morally inferior human beings than is the case today. . . . We should literally replace all factors responsible for selection in a natural and free life. . . . In prehistoric times of humanity, selection for endurance, heroism, social usefulness, etc. was made solely by *hostile* outside factors. This role must be assumed by a human organization; otherwise, humanity will, for lack of selective factors, be annihilated by the degenerative phenomena that accompany domestication."

Any ideology—which means any overriding commitment to an integrated set of intellectual assumptions and arguments—can easily lead to an arrogant disdain for other points of view. When this becomes allied with a political capacity and willingness to deal aggressively with obstacles to achieving those ideological goals, terrible violence can follow.

The ideology need not be based on genetic or other biological assumptions. Other repressive and violent regimes have been established based on ideologies that have rejected a biological basis for psychopathology in favor of a thoroughgoing sociocultural explanation. The Soviet Union under Stalin and Cambodia under Pol Pot come immediately to mind. With an unquestioning conviction about their "scientific" understanding of the profound effects of economic and political forces on

all sorts of human experiences, including psychopathology, these regimes rejected modern genetics in favor of a belief that seemed to be
more compatible with their political ideology (Lysenkoism).

Like the Nazis, they implemented policies that caused incalculable
suffering to innocent people, justifying their actions by appealing to the
need for radical solutions specified by their particular ideology. Instead
of the "sanctity of the volk," the "dictatorship of the proletariat" became
the justification for terror and murder. It is worth noting that, like the
Nazis, the Communists also found it useful to use psychiatrists to accomplish political ends and rationalized this practice on the basis of
theories derived from "scientific Marxism-Leninism."

All scientifc theories and ideas can lead to important consequences
in the way we think about and act with regard to ourselves, our world,
our relationships with others, our philosophies, our religions. The biological approach to psychiatry, like any other approach, can lead to
undesirable consequences. Narrowly understood and implemented, it
can lead to an approach to patients that is insensitive, lacking in em-
pathy, and exclusively technological. Many are concerned that the approach to patients in general medicine already shows this undesirable
effect. But it need not be this way. The broad view of biology presented
here includes the indiviudal's subjective experiences (including goals,
concerns, and needs) and sociocultural context (including family circumstances and other support systems) that must be taken into consideration for the fullest understanding of illness and optimal treatment.
This is true for the rest of medicine as it is for psychiatry.

We must understand also that nonbiological conceptual systems applied to psychiatry may have undesirable consequences. The hypothesis
of the schizophrenigenic mother, already discussed, has led to much
guilt, misery, and anger on the part of parents and others who have had
to cope with the many facets of the illness over many years. The emphasis on dynamic psychotherapy has contributed, certainly inadver-
tently, to the abandonment of many severely ill psychiatric patients because they were not considered "good psychotherapy" cases. Finally,
"labeling theory" deprives patients and their families of the sympathy,
consideration, and special treatment afforded to other sick people and
their families. All approaches can lead to unanticipated "side effects."
This is true for treatments as well as for conceptual systems.

5

Psychotherapy

Psychotherapy and the Medical Model

A frequently voiced concern about the application of the medical model to psychiatric disorders has to do with its implications for psychotherapy. The many and varied definitions of psychotherapy, different views as to specific skills and training required for its practice, differing ideas about the effects of psychotherapy, and the large number of schools of psychotherapy (Guze 1988, Karasu 1977) inevitably mean that the implications for psychotherapy of the model will vary according to the way psychotherapy is conceptualized and characterized.

The practice of psychotherapy seems to be flourishing (Karasu 1977, 1986, 1989, 1990), although its place in psychiatric practice varies widely. For some psychiatrists, and for most other mental health practitioners, it continues to be the defining activity of their professional lives. For others it plays a much less central role. There are at least three reasons for this variation in the role of psychotherapy in professional practice.

The most obvious is related to the introduction of modern psychopharmacologic agents into psychiatric practice. Since psychiatrists are the only mental health practitioners who are legally permitted to prescribe psychoactive medications, only among psychiatrists might this therapeutic approach displace psychotherapy from its dominant position in practice. (It is very interesting, however, that some clinical psychologists and even a few nurse-practitioners have been working hard to persuade various state legislatures to permit their professions to write prescriptions for psychoactive medications. More will be said about this important matter later.)

The second factor has to do with economics: partly as a result of the development of modern psychoactive drugs, but mainly because of rapidly changing economic and organizational circumstances of all medical practice, some psychiatrists have delegated or referred to other mental health practitioners responsibility for carrying out psychotherapy with their patients, retaining the more "medical" responsibilities of prescribing drugs and monitoring clinical progress. This strategy is designed to maximize income because it is less time consuming than psychotherapy and because nonpsychiatric mental health specialists in general charge less for psychotherapy than psychiatrists and thus place psychiatrists at a competitive disadvantage in today's cost containment environment.

While these two factors exert tremendous influence on current psychiatric practice, it is the third factor that may prove in the long run to be most important in shaping the way psychiatrists conceptualize the place of psychotherapy in their practices. This has to do with two different views of the goals, methods, and expectations of psychotherapy (Guze 1988).

Assumptions About Psychotherapy

According to the first view, we can learn about the etiology of our patients' disorders from their communications. More specifically, this approach to psychotherapy is predicated on the assumption that the psychotherapeutic process offers the only valid basis for laying bare the nexus of psychological forces that are etiologically responsible for the patient's illness. Obviously, this approach assumes that the various disorders being treated psychotherapeutically have such a nexus of psychological factors operating at the etiological level and that these can be correctly recognized through psychotherapy.

A very clear restatement of the assumptions underlying etiology-based psychotherapy was made by an experienced teacher of such psychotherapy at the Menninger Clinic, Glen O. Gabbard: "The psychodynamic approach asserts that we are consciously confused and unconsciously controlled. We go through our lives believing we have freedom of choice, but we are actually far more restricted than we think—we are characters living out a script written by the unconscious. Our choice of marital partners, our vocational interests, even our leisure-time pursuits are not randomly selected; they are shaped by unconscious forces in dynamic relationship with one another" (Gabbard 1990a, 1990b).

This says nothing about psychopathology, but Gabbard makes it clear

later that he includes psychiatric disorders among "unconsciously controlled" experiences. He adds two qualifications: "The principle of psychic
determinism, although certainly a bedrock notion, requires two dis-
claimers. First, unconscious factors do not determine all behaviors or
symptoms. For example, when a patient with Alzheimer's dementia for-
gets the name of his or her spouse, it probably is not unconsciously
determined. Or, when a patient with partial complex seizures ritualist-
ically buttons and unbuttons his or her shirt during the aura of the
seizure, the symptom can likely be attributed to an irritable focus of the
temporal lobe. The dynamic psychiatrist's task is to sort out which
symptoms and behaviors can be explained by dynamic factors" (Gabbard 1990b, page 8).

Gabbard proposes no satisfactory guidelines for making such judgments, however. Nor does he offer any reason for making an allowance
for patients with neurological but not psychiatric disorders, such as
schizophrenia or manic-depressive illness. One is tempted to ask how
he might decide in a patient with cerebrovascular disease whether a
particular behavior should be attributed to the neurological condition
rather than to psychodynamic undercurrents.

His second disclaimer is "derived from experience with patients who
refuse to change their behavior, claiming that they are passive victims
of unconscious forces. Within the concept of psychic determinism, there
is room for choice. While it may be more restricted than we like to
think, conscious intention to change can be an influential factor in
recovery from symptoms. The dynamic psychiatrist must be wary of
patients who justify remaining ill by claiming to be victims of unconscious forces beyond their control." Here again he provides no specific
guides for recognizing this distinction.

The etiological model of psychotherapy is inherently dramatic and
appealing. By dealing with etiology, it seems to offer the best possibility
that the patient can be cured and that future relapses can be prevented.
Its success, however, depends directly on the validity of the etiological
hypotheses. To the extent that these are in error, the ultimate justification for the psychotherapy is seriously undermined.

The second broad view of psychotherapy has been characterized as
rehabilitative (Guze 1988, Guze and Murphy 1963). It is a more limited approach with a less powerful conceptual framework. It requires no
assumptions about the etiology of the disorders being treated. As with

psychotherapy predicated upon an etiological framework, the patient's symptoms, personality, and life circumstances are reviewed and assessed. Attitudes, emotions, perceptions, strengths, weaknesses, expectations, and relationships are explored, characterized, and discussed. The aim is to help the patient understand himself or herself better and function more effectively, with less discomfort and less disability, even when little is known about the reasons for the patient's illness or how the patient's personality developed.

The main difference between these two psychotherapeutic strategies is in their contrasting approaches to etiology. But the raw material in both approaches is basically the same. It consists of observations and communications by the patient, therapist, and others (spouses, parents, friends, nurses).

The patient's communications may take several forms: spontaneous conversing with the therapist, answering questions, verbalizing free associations, describing dreams, responding to psychological tests, and so on. The therapist observes the patient's approach to the therapist and the therapeutic situation, notes and considers the form and content of the patient's statements, and assesses the patient's emotional and cognitive state. The therapist expresses any need for more information and suggests possible ways of thinking about the various responses from the patient.

Interpretations in Psychotherapy

At the operational level, the two basic approaches to psychotherapy are reflected in the nature of the interpretations offered by the psychotherapists. It is here that different assumptions about etiology are most likely to be evident. Therapists whose psychotherapeutic approaches are based on etiologic assumptions shape their comments and interpretations so as to suggest causal connections, while those skeptical about such assumptions avoid etiological interpretations. At the same time, the wide range of etiologic interpretations, reflecting the many "schools" of psychotherapy (Karasu 1986), raises fundamental issues of validity about all interpretations. We need to consider how we are to judge the correctness of all interpretations and choose between them. When they embody etiological hypotheses connecting overt psychopathology with putative causal factors, we need to consider the direction of causality. When confronted with such pairings, we must ask "which is cause and which is effect?"

While the validity of interpretation is ultimately the most important concern, the closely related issue of reliability is also relevant. It has been suggested that the reliability of an interpretation is inversely related to the "depth" of the interpretation. This is speculative but it does seem plausible that higher reliability is achievable when deducing from the patient's words, gestures, and facial expression that he or she is depressed, angry, or suspicious than it is to deduce from associations and dreams that the patient is expressing "unconscious hostility to the introjected mother" or "defending against unconscious homosexual impulses."

Yet is is this sort of interpretation, dealing with "deeply repressed" unconscious forces, that gives etiological theories of psychotherapy their special attraction and power. This is why questions about reliability and validity of interpretation are so important and why the absence of systematic, controlled studies constitutes such a serious weakness.

It is possible to achieve high levels of reliability in psychotherapy research if the therapists agree beforehand about the criteria to use for making any interpretation and if they are willing to practice sufficiently to reduce ambiguity and uncertainty. Reasonable reliability is feasible, for example, if everyone agrees to interpret all elongated structures in dreams as symbols of the penis or all frightening dreams involving attacks by other males as symbols of latent homosexuality. It would also be possible to achieve agreement about ambiguous dreams using explicit algorithms. Thus, everyone could reach the same interpretation about a dream in which the sex of the attacker is not clear or in which the elongated structure is imbedded in a large number of similar structures (what might look like a grove of trees) so that its identity is obscured. In such cases, it would not matter whether or nor the interpretation is correct or incorrect; a satisfactory level of reliability would be possible. The point is obvious, however, that such reliability by itself would not be useful. Reliability is important only when it can be coupled to validity.

Closely related to questions of reliability, but of greater import, is the likelihood that a therapist's interpretations may actually reflect his or her own assumptions and expectations, thus constituting "suggestion" rather than a disinterested and objective response to the patient's communications. It is difficult to rule out the possibility that all interpretations are vulnerable to such distortions. This is reflected in the old and cynical adage that every therapist finds in patients just what his or her orientation leads the therapist to expect.

In his detailed critique of psychoanalysis, Adolph Grünbaum, a professor of philosophy at the University of Pittsburgh, reminds us that Freud tried seriously to deal with criticism about the powerful effects of suggestion within the psychoanalytic process, but he concludes that Freud's efforts were not successful (Grünbaum 1984, pages 133–135). According to Grünbaum, Freud thought that three kinds of clinical findings could be preserved from such distortion: "the products of 'free' association, the patient's assent to analytic interpretations that he or she had initially resisted, and memories recovered from early life." But Grünbaum disagrees because the therapist will inevitably show more or less interest in different communications from the patient, which in turn will influence the patient's subsequent responses. Thus, if the therapist pays more attention to things the patient says that are consistent with the therapist's assumptions than to those that are not consistent, the patient may well respond accordingly.

Donald Spence, an experienced psychologist and psychotherapist, has also written about suggestion and the reliability and validity of psychotherapeutic interpretations (Spence 1982, 1987). He has articulated these interrelated concerns so clearly and fully that it is worth quoting him at some length: "Freud, the first psychoanalyst, was also one of the first great synthesizers. He was a master at taking pieces of the patient's associations, dreams, and memories and weaving them into a coherent pattern that is compelling, persuasive, and seemingly complete, a pattern that allows us to make important discoveries about the patient's life and to make sense out of previously random happenings. . . . Freud made us aware of the persuasive power of a coherent narrative—in particular, the way in which an aptly chosen reconstruction can fill the gap between two apparently unrelated events and, in the process, make sense out of nonsense. There seems no doubt that a well-constructed story possesses a kind of narrative truth that is real and immediate and carries an important significance for the therapeutic change" (Spence 1982, pages 21–22).

The distinction between narrative and historical truth is at the heart of Spence's thoughtful critique of psychotherapeutic interpretations. How closely does what we hear or bring out during psychotherapy reflect actual events in the patient's life as they happened or the patient's reconstruction of these experiences guided by the therapist's theoretical assumptions, or the patient's expectations based upon cultural beliefs and indoctrination? Spence elaborates: "To an extent that has not been appreciated up to now, the narrative tradition has turned us all into searchers after meaning and, to a significant degree, has prevented us from following Freud's rule of listening with evenly hovering attention. . . . The narrative tradition has had an important influence on our literature as well. . . . Because the raw data have no secure place in this tradition, they tend to be left out . . . streamlined case reports have tended to take the place of the original data, and our basic observations, until very recently, have tended to disappear once they were uttered. As a result, the path from observation to theory can never be retraced; thus we have no way to confirm or disconfirm an observation, much less combine all observations into a new formulation. . . . The model of the patient as unbiased reporter and the analyst as unbiased listener suggests the kind of naive realism that is hard to imagine, harder to practice, and runs counter to everything we have learned about the way we come to understand the world. . . . the psychoanalytic literature makes no provision for alternative explanations of the same data. A case report is presented as a record of the facts, not as an interpretation of some of the data; this convention is a natural consequence of the assumption that the analyst functions as a largely unbiased reporter" (pages 22–25).

Spence comes to the conclusion: "Coupling the narrative tradition with a Freudian model leads to a failure to distinguish between two kinds of truth. . . . Narrative truth is confused with historical truth, and the very coherence of an account may lead us to believe that we are making contact with an actual happening. Moreover, what is effective for a given patient in a particular hour (the narrative truth of an interpretation) may be mistakenly attributed to its historical foundations" (page 27). Or, to put it another way, "Interpretations are persuasive . . . not because of their evidential value but because of their rhetorical appeal; conviction emerges because the fit is good, not because we have necessarily made contact with the past. . . . If we confuse narrative truth with historical . . . truth, we will never make the necessary distinction, and our theory will never rise much above the level of metaphor" (pages 32–33).

These are severe criticisms, but they are consistent with the following observations other leading psychotherapists have also made. In a symposium on the efficacy of psychotherapy (Myers 1984), Robert Michels, a nationally recognized psychoanalyst and professor of psychiatry at Cornell University, offered a perspective that also challenges the historical truth of patients' communications. "In June of 1882 Breuer stopped his treatment of Anna O, fled from it as a matter of fact, and in November of 1882 . . . he told Freud about the case and psychoanalysis began. [For the next fifteen years,] the basic model of psychoanalysis and of the genesis of psychopathology was that some traumatic event, rapidly recognized to be an event in the childhood of the patient, had caused the pathology and that recovery of the memory of that event in the treatment was curative" (pages 83–85).

At this point, Michels presents a view that is controversial. Not all psychoanalysts believe that Freud's "discovery" was correct, but many others do share Michels' view: "Freud made a dramatic discovery in 1897. He discovered, as he reported to his correspondent friend Fliess, that his patients had been telling him things that weren't true and the traumatic events that they described to him and that he had assumed were etiologic had often, if not generally, not occurred. They had simply been the results of the patients' imaginations. A minor figure would have hoped that no one else found out the same thing. A great figure would have reported his error and retracted his theory. A genius like Freud did neither of those. He reported his error but maintained his theory, pointing out that this was an even more important discovery because it meant that the traumatic experiences which he had thought reflected something about the adult's behavior with children, in fact, told us something about the mind of the growing child, that the trauamtic events of childhood which were pathogenic were really fantasies rather than events in the life of the child. . . . central to that notion is that what was pathogenic for the child in psychoanalytic theory was not the way that he was treated by his parents, was not the way he was understood or misunderstood or traumatized, and that treating him well can't be curative because treating him badly was not the problem in the first place. . . . Was Freud wrong in 1897?"

Michels' position raises serious questions about the historical truth of some of the things patients tell psychotherapists. There is certainly an important difference between a fantasy and an historical event.

At the same symposium with Michels, another highly regarded practitioner and investigator of psychotherapy and a professor of psychiatry at Johns Hopkins University, Dr. Jerome Frank, stressed the potential for influencing the patient's verbalizations during psychotherapy (Myers 1984, pages 89–90). "I really want to introduce another note of doubt or caution into all of this, a very fundamental one, and that's the validity of the evidential base on which all psychoanalytic theory rests. It rests on patient's reports to the analyst about what happened. Now, Freud thought that his method would yield objective data, because the analyst is simply a mirror and the patient is allowed to freely associate without being influenced by the analyst. By now it is perfectly clear that this is an extremely powerful influencing situation. In fact, it is very analogous to one of the most successful forms of brainwashing, that is, the prisoner is asked to confess, but he is never told whether his confession is right or not. He is just told to keep on confessing and eventually something good will happen. This is what you really have in an analytic situation—where the patient comes to the analyst because he is in distress. He's like a prisoner in that sense. He's looking to the analyst for relief and the analyst doesn't give him relief, he just says, go on talking, go on free associating and eventually you will get relief. But this creates a situation that I remember when I was in analysis, where the analysand becomes extremely sensitive to the slightest cues to what interests the analyst and what doesn't. I remember seeing the analyst's foot waving out of the corner of my eye, noting when he seemed to be writing; things like this. All the time the analyst is subtly guiding what the analysand comes up with. The essential point is that this can lead to false memory. This was shown in brainwashing. Very often the prisoner would finally confess to things he really thought had happened which had never happened. So, I would raise the question about the whole basis for our theories here."

Marshall Edelson (1988), another psychoanalyst and professor of psychiatry at Yale University, in a book also concerned with the validity of what comes up in psychotherapy, observes that psychoanalysis, "despite the historicism of many of its theoretical formulations, is not a historical science, but is instead a science of the symbolizing activity of the mind.

Psychoanalysis cannot be concerned merely with the recovery of the actual historical past. As a method it is not suitable for the study of actual events. A patient may refer to what is apparently the same event at different times and in different contexts during a psychoanlaysis. At these different times and in these different contexts, presentations of the event, its elements and properties, differ. Details, emphases, conceptions of the event and of its significance, and the attitudes and feelings aroused by or associated with the event, differ. The very history of the patient seems to change as he reconstructs it during different periods of a psychoanalysis. What the event and its elements and properties mean, what the patient, using 'actualities' as material, made and makes of them, changes. If a history is revived, it is the history of the acts of the patient's mind, creating through time his symbolic representations of his conceptions of the past, present, and future 'reality.'

"We may or may not infer an actual event at that imaginary point where a patient's symbolic representations of that event seem to converge. But that actual event as an entity is not knowable through, and cannot be investigated by, psychoanalysis. The pathogens exorcised by psychoanalysis are not physiological processes or historical situations but symbolic representations of conceptions of such processes and situations and transformations of these symbolic representations: mental shades, memories, fantasies. Not reality but symbolic representations of conceptions of reality. Not organism but symbolic representations of conceptions of the body. Not object-relations but symbolic representations of conceptions of objects and kinds of relations to them. Between stimulus and response, between event and behavior, falls the act of the mind. It is the creation of the symbol, the 'poem of the act of the mind' that is the object of study in psychoanalysis" (pages 19–20).

These quotations from Grünbaum, Spence, Michels, Frank, and Edelson embody two questions: the validity of the patient's communciations and the validity of the therapist's interpretations. From varying perspectives and in different ways, each of these authors raises doubts about their validity. We are left with considerable uncertainty about the historical truth of many things that come up in the therapeutic situation. We are equally uncertain about the degree to which therapists influence what patients report to them, shaping and guiding their stories and reports so that they are consistent with the assumptions and beliefs of the therapists.

In addition, insufficient emphasis has been placed on the powerful impact of cultural beliefs on patient's communications. Psychoanalytic ideas are deeply imbedded in our culture, through the impact of books, films, TV, and teaching in schools at all levels. This has typically happened without a corresponding critique of the evidence upon which the theory is based. It would certainly be expected, therefore, that many patients, and perhaps most, would communicate at least some thoughts, feelings, and memories that seem to be consistent with their understanding of what is expected of them, according to the theory. In other words, cultural beliefs can serve as a source of suggestion and bias that may greatly influence what takes place in psychotherapy.

Psychotherapeutic Interpretations and Causal Direction

The validity of psychotherapeutic interpretations faces another major hurdle: the direction of causality (Guze 1988). Let us assume that it proves feasible, with much effort, to achieve a reasonable level of agreement as to the meaning of what the patient says in psychotherapy and that we can set aside questions about reliability and suggestion. Furthermore, let's also set aside questions about the specificity of interpretations discussed in Chapter 1. The question that would still have to be addressed is whether it would be possible to distinguish between two alternative possibilities: the psychologically meaningful experience, or the symbol of such experience, identified in the interpretation, could be the *cause* of the patient's disorder or it could be the *effect* of the disorder.

From their psychotherapy sessions, the therapist may conclude that the patient shows a consistent and characteristic pattern of responding to the manifold demands and challenges of life. This pattern may be revealed in the patient's expectations, perceptions, emotions, and in what are called defense mechanisms. The therapist may try to help the patient recognize these patterns, appreciate the way they affect relations with others, and try to modify those patterns that the patient regards as disabling. The patient's pattern of reacting to the therapist and the therapeutic situation (transference) may be used as a tool for identifying and describing the patient's emotions and behavioral patterns and as a vehicle for efforts to change.

The patient's history may be explored for indications concerning the onset and evolution of these patterns, which may appear traceable to earlier periods in the patient's life. The same patterns may be encountered in the patient's spontaneous talk, free associations, dreams, and responses to projective tests. But it is clear that the psychotherapeutic situation does not permit the therapist to determine which causal factors—interpersonal, situational, cultural, or physiological—were responsible for the development of the presenting disorder or the adaptive patterns of behavior. Of course, we may speculate; we may look for supporting evidence in other aspects of the patient's history; and we may search for similar experiences in other patients. But finally we must accept that the therapeutic situation has limitations that cannot be transcended. These have already been noted: the therapeutic situation cannot get around the problems of therapist bias and suggestion, patient expectation, and direction of causality. Our theories can only be tested through experiments, whether designed by humans or by nature.

During psychotherapy with patients suffering from any clinical disorder, certain ideas, feelings, moods, attitudes, fears, and desires may be observed and their causal relationship to the presenting problem considered, but it is not possible to tell whether these psychological states are causal or consequential. Simple coincidence may be excluded if other patients with the same disorder have the same psychological experiences, as long as the observations are controlled for potentially confounding variables. But even these findings do not allow us to distinguish between the two directions of causality. This requires experimentation.

If we were to speculate that schizophrenia results from some as yet unidentified neurobiological abnormalities, it seems likely that the abnormalities would not only lead to the overt clinical manifestations of the disorder, such as delusions and hallucinations, but would also profoundly affect the content and tone of free assocations and dreams. The interpretations derived from the dreams and free associations of schizophrenic patients, rather than identifying causes of the overt condition, would merely be recognizing less overt manifestations of it.

In summary, there is little scientific basis for the assumption that psychotherapy serves as *the vehicle to uncover the etiology of psychiatric disorders.* Thus, if the etiological hypotheses underlying etiology-based psychotherapy are flawed, the scientific status of such psychotherapy is in doubt.

Rehabilitative Psychotherapy

The rehabilitative view of psychotherapy (Guze 1988, Guze and Murphy 1963) appears to avoid such scientific risk. It requires no assumptions concerning etiology or pathogenesis, and it may be implemented through a variety of techniques. In fact, many current approaches to psychotherapy, including cognitive therapy, interpersonal therapy, and behavior modification, can all be subsumed under the rehabilitation umbrella. Even a non-etiological approach to psychodynamic psychotherapy, in which the therapist offers no etiologically significant interpretations, can be included under the same rubric.

Rehabilitative psychotherapy is entirely compatiable with the medical model in psychiatry, because it is independent of etiology and thus faces no difficulties about diagnostic specificity. It may be used in a wide range of conditions of presumably diverse etiology and pathogenesis. It permits the therapist to take into consideration many potentially relevant factors in an attempt to help the patient shift the balance toward a more satisfactory outcome.

An analogy with another area of medicine may be useful. Physical therapy and rehabilitation medicine are similarly indicated for a wide range of conditions, including orthopedic, neurologic, cardiac, rheumatic, and other disorders. The treatments are largely independent of the wide range of etiologies. Optimally, the treatments are designed to take into consideration the patient's age, strength, education, personality, previous skills, motivation, social and family circumstances, all with the goal of alleviating the physical disability.

The strategic focus in rehabilitative psychotherapy is on helping the patient better understand the presenting illness or problem and on developing approaches for minimizing the difficulties or disabilities associated with the illness or problem. Requiring no assumptions concerning etiology, it encourages shifts of attention to the individual's specific circumstances and situation. Rehabilitative psychotherapy is relatively nonspecific regarding the illness or disorder, but specific concerning the patient's circumstances and personality.

The goals may be summarized in a number of questions that the patient and therapist, together, try to answer. These include: What are the aspects of treatment (including costs and side effects) that must be understood and agreed to? What are the implications of the expected course and prognosis of the presenting condition? What are the patient's strengths and weaknesses as they bear on his or her adaptation to this condition? What are the patient's circumstances, including support systems and responsibilities? What are the patient's adaptive style and coping mechanisms? How are these affected by the illness? Are there identifiable patterns in the patient's approach to people and problems?

The rationale behind these and similar questions is that they may help the patient recognize circumstances and coping patterns that are less than optimal and consider various ways of improving them. When such a process of psychotherapy is successful, the patient may feel better, suffer less disability, and cope more effectively. In these ways, psychotherapy can be an important part of the treatment of patients with a wide variety of clinical conditions.

There is extensive clinical experience upon which to draw concerning different ways of helping patients learn to think about their illnesses and associated problems. Experienced clinicians know much about ways to interview patients and discuss these difficulties constructively. A good deal of this knowledge is not systematic or specific, but this can be changed as more psychotherapists identify the questions to be addressed in focused, systematic studies.

Clearly, the medical model is not incompatible with an acceptance of the importance of psychotherapy in psychiatric practice. Good psychiatry, like good medicine in general, must involve much more than making a diagnosis and prescribing appropriate medications. There is little dispute among experienced clinicians that psychologically significant events and emotional reactions can affect the body's physiological state. Nor is there any dispute that discussions about their clinical problems and life circumstances can be helpful to patients. Most sick persons need and want such discussions. Where agreement is much less likely is with the important matter, already discussed, concerning the limitations in establishing causal linkages during psychotherapy.

Psychotherapy: Meaning of Illness and How It Helps

Finally, any discussion of psychotherapy and what can be expected from it must consider the important issue of the meaning of illness. This question of meaning is closely related to the issue of narrative truth. Narrative truth and the meaning of illness are derived, at least indirectly, from the philosophical tradition of hermeneutics. This tradition holds "that we cannot do justice to actions as meaningful while we seek a naturalistic or scientific analysis of them and that the aim of social science [specifically including psychology] must be intelligibility, whereas its means should be interpretation" (Rosenberg 1988). Efforts to understand events and experiences from this perspective of "meaning" are directed to the formulation of plausible and coherent stories that serve as the basis for narrative truth.

Such stories, in the form of interpretations during psychotherapy, offer "insight" that may have therapeutic value even when they have no scientific basis (Spence 1982). Thus, some features of psychotherapy add meaning to the patient's condition, whatever its nature. Perhaps the desire to give illness meaning is related to the nearly universal need for understanding and explanation, especially when experiences are painful or life-threatening. But we must recognize clearly that such meaning is quite different from what physicians have always understood by etiology.

To summarize: psychotherapy can provide much needed emotional support, the chance to discuss and understand one's self better, an opportunity to consider the meaning of one's illness and related experiences, a safe and protected situation in which to explore various options and possibilities that take into consideration one's personal attributes and circumstances, and a special environment in which frustrations and anger may be freely expressed. The psychotherapeutic process can also lead to hypotheses about etiology, but it does not allow for the critical testing of such hypotheses. Psychotherapy offers no way to control for the preexisting assumptions of the therapist or the patient, nor for the effect on the patient's communications of the therapist's interpretations and suggestions. And, significantly, the psychotherapeutic process does not allow one to determine the causal relationships between phenomena of interest considered during psychotherapy and the patient's clinical problems. Nevertheless, psychotherapy, especially when based upon a rehabilitation strategy, is fully compatible with the medical model. Only those who believe that psychotherapy is the best path to identifying etiology are likely to object seriously to the basic arguments presented here.

6

Philosophical Issues

This chapter deals with important issues that psychiatrists must consider, at least implicitly, as they think about the nature and significance of psychiatric problems and disorders. These include: causality, teleology, the relationship between the mind and the brain, reductionism, free will, consciousness, the meaning of illness, and a number of important ethical matters. These topics have been the focus of extensive and highly specialized study and analysis by many experienced philosophers (Hundert 1989). The emphasis here will be on the implications for these philosophical issues of observations and experiences from psychiatric practice and thinking.

Causality

Medical thinking has always incorporated the idea of cause, and causal hypotheses have been inseparably linked to treatment strategies. Because psychiatry deals with motivation, goals, and intention, subjects of great complexity from a causal perspective, psychiatrists are brought face to face with certain philosophical concerns linked to questions about cause.

Physicians have tended to divide causes into three types: those that are necessary and sufficient, those that are necessary but not sufficient, and those that are predisposing or facilitating but neither necessary nor sufficient.

Necessary and sufficient causes are uncommon in medicine. Recognized examples seem largely to be genes that produce illnesses that follow Mendelian patterns of inheritance with more or less complete penetrance (Scriver et al. 1989). Phenylketonuria, sickle-cell anemia, certain

forms of color blindness, certain forms of cancer, and certain hyperli-
pidemias are illnesses with such causes. Though, in the case of phenylketonuria, ubiquitous dietary phenylalanine is also necessary. The
number of such conditions is increasing with research progress and is
likely to continue increasing, but at the present time, they constitute a
small proportion of all illnesses. Another kind of necessary and sufficient causes consists of highly toxic chemicals that produce illness in all
individuals exposed to the threshold amount. In all these circumstances, the presence of the cause invariably results in illness.

For most illnesses where a necessary cause has been identified, the
cause has proven to be necessary but not sufficient. The most widely
recognized among this group of causes are infectious organisms.

Tuberculosis is a classical example. To produce tuberculosis, the tu-
bercle bacillus is necessary. But being exposed to the organism is not
sufficient to cause the illness. It has long been known that exposure to
the bacillus, manifested by a positive tuberculin test, generally produces
overt illness only in a minority of exposed individuals. Other factors are
important: those that modify the virulence of the bacillus (generally
through genetic changes in the bacillus) or those that modify the resistance of the host. Among the latter are malnutrition, alcoholism, other
substance abuse, various socioeconomic variables such as poverty and
overcrowding, and genetic predisposition. The situation is similar for
other infectious disorders: exposure to the infectious agent is generally
not sufficient to produce illness.

Another example of a cause that is insufficient but necessary may be
seen in alcoholism. As with infectious illnesses named after the infectious agent, alcoholism is identified by the chemical substance to which
the individual is exposed. And, as with infections, not everyone exposed
to alcohol develops alcoholism. Other factors are involved, including
genetic, cultural, and social influences.

These influences, which have been demonstrated repeatedly to affect
the risk of developing an infection or of becoming an alcoholic, illustrate what is meant by modifying or facilitating factors. They are not
necessary causes because the particular disorder is possible in the absence of any one of them, so far as we can tell today. Neither are they
sufficient causes because they are incapable of producing the illness in
the absence of the necessary cause. Of course, it is possible that for
some disorders, perhaps even for most, it will turn out that there is

more than one necessary cause. For instance, there have been reports that two separate gene mutations are needed for at least some cases of retinoblastoma (Dryja et al. 1989).

Facilitating or modifying factors are often called "risk factors." Their role in many disorders, most strikingly with regard to coronary heart disease, has received a great deal of public attention. Few people have not heard about obesity, elevated cholesterol levels, smoking, high blood pressure, a positive family history, and type A personality as influencing the risk of developing coronary atherosclerosis. But the fact that individuals may develop cardiovascular disorders in the absence of any of these risk factors is much less well appreciated. Nonetheless, recognizing and attempting to combat these risk factors can apparently help reduce the burden of coronary heart disease, even though a necessary cause has not yet been identified for the great majority of cases.

Tobacco as a risk factor for lung cancer provides another opportunity for this preventive strategy. The evidence relating smoking, and especially cigarette smoking, to the risk of lung cancer is very strong. At the same time, it is evident that some cases of lung cancer (a small percentage) occur in the absence of smoking. And, also important, only a minority of cigarette smokers develop lung cancer despite many years of smoking. Nevertheless, there is strong evidence that the risk of lung cancer can be reduced if cigarette smoking is curtailed.

Distinctions among causal categories as necessary and sufficient, necessary but not sufficient, and neither necessary nor sufficient (risk factors) are subject to the findings of new studies. It is conceivable that individual causal factors will be reclassified as more is learned. This may in turn lead to reclassifying the disorders themselves, based upon differential causal patterns. For example, it is well recognized that only about twenty-five percent of schizophrenia is associated with the same disorder in first-degree relatives; thus the putative gene(s) can only be considered a risk factor at present. But if the idea that schizophrenia can be divided into a familial form and a nonfamilial form is ultimately supported by the identification of a relevant gene(s) associated with the familial form, this gene(s) will be designated as a necessary cause for the familial subtype. In other words, the classification of causes is not immutable; it is subject to revision as knowledge increases.

The failure to find single necessary and sufficient causes for most illnesses thus far has led to the concept of multicausality. While sensible, this view can have adverse side effects because it is not always emphasized sufficiently how important it is to establish the role of *each putative cause through well-designed, controlled studies.* Ignoring the need for multiple controls in which all the factors suspected of influencing the risk of developing a given disorder are studied risks the easy acceptance of plausible hypotheses without proper scientific foundation. And it can often lead to the belief that the causal factors are different for every individual case of a particular disorder.

Of course, there is no logical requirement that there be a necessary cause for each illness. Some illnesses may result from such a large range of different causes that no two cases have the same causal pattern. In such circumstances, however, it would be impossible to establish the causal connections in any single case. The situation would be indistinguishable from a state in which no causal hypothesis could be tested and established as valid. The study of cause assumes common denominators. Emphasizing the uniqueness of the causal pattern in each case becomes scientifically sterile.

Related to the concept of multicausality is the concept of "contingent causes." This concept has been proposed to deal with unpredictable happenings that individuals and even species experience and that are proposed, *in retrospect,* to explain otherwise puzzling and surprising responses. Stephen J. Gould (1989) has insisted on the central role that "contingency" plays in "historical science," including paleontology. He argues that the value of studying the Burgess Shale (a wonderful discovery of Cambrian fossils in western Canada that raises many fascinating and important questions about evolution) "lies in its affirmation of history as the chief determinant of life's directions."

After reviewing these fossil findings Gould writes that they are "rooted in contingency. . . . The modern order [of species] was not guaranteed by basic laws (natural selection, mechanical superiority in anatomical design), or even by lower-level generalities of ecology or evolutionary theory. The modern order is largely a product of contingency."

Gould is fully aware that all scientific hypotheses depend upon "secure testability," by which he means that they must be supported by the preponderance of empirical evidence, but also recognizes that "historical explanations are distinct from conventional experimental results in many ways." He clearly knows that the "issue of verification by repetition does not arise because we are trying to account for uniqueness of detail that cannot, both by laws of probability and time's arrow of irreversibility, occur together again. We do not attempt to interpret the complex events of narrative by reducing them to simple consequences of natural law; historical events do not, of course, violate any general principle of matter and motion, but their occurrence lies in the realm of contingent detail."

Gould's argument about the centrality of contingency in evolution supports his strong belief that evolutionary history is in no way goal-directed. He welcomes the evidence that evolution is not necessarily a matter of growing complexity of species leading to ever "higher" forms. He derives great satisfaction from the conclusion that it was not inevitable that homo sapiens would develop. He finds it exciting and even reassuring that contingency and accident play such powerful roles in evolution as well as in life in general.

Gould is certainly correct as far as he goes. We are all aware that life is a matter of contingencies that *may* shape our experiences and determine much about our existence. And many may share Gould's seemingly perverse satisfaction in the evidence that we are not here to fulfill some hidden but great purpose. There is something exhilarating and brave about facing such conclusions. But it does not tell us how to evaluate any particular hypothesis concerning the role of contingency in the cause of any specific experience or reaction of a particular species or organism. Gould offers no help in distinguishing between contingency and simple ignorance of why certain things happened.

His own words reveal what the problems are in validating hypotheses in historical science. "Historical explanation takes the form of narrative: E, the phenomenon to be explained, arose because D came before, preceded by C, B, and A. If any of these earlier stages had not occurred, or had transpired in a different way, then E would not exist (or would be present in a substantially altered form, E', requiring a different explanation). Thus E makes sense and can be explained rigorously as the outcome of A through D. But no law of nature enjoined E; any variant E' arising from an altered set of antecedents would have been equally explicable, though massively different in form and effect." One need not have had much experience in testing hypotheses to appreciate instantly the problems involved in testing the links between so many things, especially if the putative causal chain involves primarily nonsystematic, idiosyncratic, personal experiences, such as occur in everyone's life, but under varying circumstances and different timing.

Gould asserts that he is "not speaking of randomness (for E had to arise, as a consequence of A through D), but the central principle of all history—*contingency*. A historical explanation does not rest on direct deductions from laws of nature, but on an unpredictable sequence of antecedent states, where any major change in any step of the sequence would have altered the final result. This final result is therefore dependent, or contingent, upon everything that came before—the unerasable and determining signature of history."

The concept of contingent causality can lead to causal hypotheses that are so difficult to test critically that they would resemble or be indistinguishable from situations where no causal hypothesis can be seriously considered. *yes - a weakness of scientific method.*

Similar views on contingency have been expressed by R. C. Lewontin, a distinguished geneticist who has long been an outspoken critic of sociobiology and of most efforts to establish causal links between heredity and human behavior (Lewontin 1990): "By its very nature, sociobiological theory is unable to cope with the extraordinary historical and cultural *contingency* of human behavior, nor with the diversity of individual behavior and its development in the course of individual life histories." We know that there is not a particularly high correlation between heredity and all aspects of behavior. The same may be said for the correlation between specific brain injuries and behavior, or between specific endocrine disorders and behavior, or even between specific cultural or familial influences and behavior.

This does not mean, however, that there are *no* regularities in such correlations or that the correlations that have been observed are of no practical or theoretical value. The absence of complete correlations means only that other factors are also involved. Some of these factors may prove to be systematic and consistent among different individuals and so become better understood in time. Others may be highly individualized, and thus contingent in the way Lewontin uses the term, so that it will be much more difficult, and perhaps impossible, to validate their causal role. The concept of contingency, as used by these authors, implies unpredictable, unsystematic, idiosyncratic events or circumstances; surely that comes close to what we mean by ignorance. For medicine, especially psychiatry, such hypotheses have been and continue to be frequently proposed as explanations concerning the etiology of many clinical conditions (Sulloway 1979).

To fill out our discussion of causality it is important to consider briefly the question of association and its relationship to cause. To distinguish between the two requires experiment. It is only through experiments that the effects of variations in hypothesized causes on the development of any particular condition can be assessed. For a great many hypothesized causes, deliberate and planned experimentation involving human subjects is not possible, whether for ethical or practical reasons. In the absence of satisfactory animal models for most psychiatrict disorders, human studies are necessary, and this nearly always means that nature's experiments must be sought out.

Satisfactory experiments of nature are often very difficult to find, however, especially when one wants to test causal hypotheses involving complex interpersonal and social experiences and relationships that begin early in life and extend over many years. There are few existing databases that offer the possibility of reconstructing such experiences and relationships in a valid and convincing way.

For example, to test hypotheses about the effects of childhood experiences on the risk of developing later illnesses, such as schizophrenia or bipolar affective disorder, it is necessary to make comparisons between people who have had a particular childhood experience and those who have not. All other potentially confounding variables must be controlled. These include all sorts of factors that might influence the development of the illness under study, such as hereditary influences, experiences during labor and delivery, general health, educational experiences, and cultural influences.

All such potentially confounding factors must be assessed before the individual's clinical status is determined (Feinstein 1967, 1985). And obviously it must be clear that the putative causal factors were operating well before the individual became ill. Accomplishing all this with a large enough sample to offer the possibility of significant findings is very difficult, especially for disorders that have relatively low prevalence rates such as schizophrenia or mania.

Because of the tremendous difficulties associated with the population-based strategy for assessing the causal role of any hypothesized experience in the development of psychiatric disorders, investigators often turn to what are called high-risk studies. This approach builds upon the recognition that many psychiatric conditions are familial. By studying other family members who are as yet free of the disorder in question, especially children of index cases, one can get by with a much smaller sample, counting on the expected increased prevalence of the condition in close relatives. Though there can be confounding variables in high risk studies, they have an additional advantage that may prove helpful in studying etiology. Periodic, regular examination of the high-risk sample makes it possible to establish more accurately when a given disorder begins. This permits a more informed approach to possibly causal experiences that antedate the onset of the disorder. Of course, such high-risk designs may not always permit one to extrapolate any findings to nonfamilial forms of the condition.

Clearly, studies of causality (etiology) are extremely difficult. This is especially true when testing hypotheses about the effects of long-term, persistent, psychosocial circumstances or of ongoing patterns of important interpersonal relationships. Inevitably, such studies will present major problems when it comes to interpreting the results. We must depend on consistent findings from different studies of different populations, and we must search for various kinds of corroborative observations. Fortunately, causal hypotheses that do not involve complex psychosocial or cultural factors are generally easier to test. It may be that after the causal role in psychiatric conditions of genetic and neurobiological factors has been established, it will be easier to test major psychosocial and cultural hypotheses. By controlling for genetic and physiological factors, the role of the psychosocial and cultural environment will become magnified and more clearly evident.

To return to strategic causal thinking, another way that scientists, especially biological scientists, have viewed the matter of cause has been to divide causes into *proximate* and *ultimate* (Mayr 1988). In discussing the cause of the migration of a warbler at his summer place in New Hampshire, Mayr lists "four equally legitimate causes for this migration: (1) *An ecological cause.* The warbler, being an insect eater, must migrate, because it would starve to death if it should try to winter in New Hampshire. (2) *A genetic cause.* The warbler has acquired a genetic constitution in the course of the evolutionary history of its species which induces it to respond appropriately to the proper stimuli from the environment. On the other hand, the screech owl, nesting right next to it, lacks this constitution and does not respond to these stimuli. As a result, it is sedentary. (3) *An intrinsic physiological cause*. The warbler flew south because its migration is tied in with photoperiodicity. It responds to the decrease in day length and is ready to migrate as soon as the number of hours of daylight have dropped below a certain level. (4) *An extrinsic physiological cause*. Finally, the warbler migrated on the 25th of August because a cold air mass, with northerly winds, passed over our area on that day. The sudden drop in temperature and the associated weather conditions affected the bird, already in a general physiological readiness for migration, so that it actually took off on that particular day."

Mayr assigns the first two causes to the *ultimate* category and the second two causes to the *proximate* category. He observes that the "functional biologist would be concerned with . . . analysis of the proximate causes, while the evolutionary biologist would be concerned with analysis of ultimate causes," adding that this "is the case with almost any biological phenomenon we might want to study. There is always a proximate set of causes and an ultimate set of causes; both have to be explained and interpreted for a complete understanding of the given phenomenon."

However, evolutionary explanations alone are rarely, if ever, satisfactory explanations for disease or ill health. Unless evolutionary explanations are tied directly to genetic and physiological knowledge of why some people get sick in certain ways while others do not, they are too vague and general to be useful in medicine. For example, the liver is an organ that evolved to meet certain needs. Obviously, a liver must be present for an individual to develop hepatitis, so that, in some sense, evolution may be offered as an explanation for the hepatitis. But without evidence for specific genetic predisposition or for specific differences in liver morphology or physiology contributing to the differential vulnerability, the evolutionary explanation is scientifically impoverished. Similarly, evolution has shaped the human brain and its mental capacities and responses, but without demonstrated connections between specific genetic contributions or physiological functions and particular psychiatric disorders, invoking evolution as a causal factor for these disorders is not illuminating.

Causality is a very complicated issue, which can be approached in many ways. In medicine generally, causality has been approached from the point of view of treatment and prevention. Physicians have been interested in causal factors that lend themselves to medical intervention. They have been inclined therefore to focus on what Mayr designated as proximate causes.

Teleology

Teleology of course refers to the idea that goals serve as causes of behavior. No discussion of causality involving living organisms can ignore the problems that stem from attributing causal power to the end result of an action, because it requires an explanation as to how a *later* event can cause an *earlier* one. Ernst Mayr has dealt with this matter as thoroughly and effectively as anyone (Mayr 1988, pages 29–31, 38–66). He reminds us that this "problem had its beginning with Aristotle's classification of causes, one of the categories being the 'final' causes. This category is based on the observation of the orderly and purposive development of the individual from the egg to the 'final' stage of the adult. Final cause has been defined as 'the cause responsible for the orderly reaching of a preconceived ultimate goal.' All goal-seeking behavior has been classified as 'teleological.' "

After dismissing previous attempts to deal with this matter that introduced "dualistic, finalistic, and vitalistic" explanations, Mayr insists that there is an acceptable answer to the question, "Where, then, is it legitimate to speak of purpose and purposiveness in nature, and where is it not?" He argues that "to this question we can now give a firm and unambiguous answer. An individual who—to use the language of the computer—has been 'programmed' can act purposefully. . . . The completely individualistic and yet also species-specific DNA program of every zygote (fertilized egg cell), which controls the development of the central and peripheral nervous systems, of the sense organs, of the hormones, of physiology and morphology, is the *program* for the behavior computer of this individual. . . . Natural selection does its best to favor the production of programs guaranteeing behavior that increase fitness." Mayr prefers the term *teleonomic* for such purposive behavior. J. Z. Young, the highly respected British physiologist presents similar views in his book entitled *Programs of the Brain* (Young 1978).

We know all too little about the anatomical or physiological characteristics of the built-in programs in humans that guide the individual's responses to experience. But the teleonomic conception of such programs offers an approach to the causes of goal-directed behavior that does not require the difficult assumption that later events can cause earlier ones.

Mind-Brain Interactions

What is the relationship between the mind and the brain or body? This vitally important question has been at the center of philosophical concern for a long time. In recent years, with new developments in biological research, especially molecular genetics and neuroscience, a renewed interest in the question is also evident among scientists and physicians (Changeaux 1985, Eccles 1980, 1989, Popper and Eccles 1977, Edelman 1987, Gazzaniga 1985, Goodman 1991, Hundert 1989, Posner 1989, Young 1987). It has fascinated and frustrated psychiatrists of all types, and it is probably correct to say that the way one thinks about mind-brain issues profoundly affects the way one thinks about psychiatry. It certainly shapes one's views on the place of neuroscience in psychiatry. If one believes that the mind is something different from the brain, then neuroscience would have little to teach psychiatrists that is pertinent to their practices. This dualism seriously undermines the validity of any serious approach to the pharmacological treatment of psychiatric conditions. How can prescribing medication do anything for mental disturbances if they are located in the mind and not in the brain where the drugs presumably act? But it is already clear that drugs do affect all sorts of mental processes and experiences. They can sedate, calm without sedation, reduce or eliminate hallucinations and delusions, diminish or eliminate obsessions and panic attacks, and modify depression and mania. And, very importantly, they can also *cause* panic attacks, depression, mania, and a variety of psychotic experiences, including hallucinations and delusions. That manipulation of the brain through pharmacological intervention can profoundly influence mental experiences is beyond question.

That mental experiences can affect all sorts of bodily processes, including brain processes, is also beyond doubt. There is a vast literature demonstrating clearly that mental experiences affect endocrine and other metabolic systems, the cardiovascular and gastrointestinal systems, the immune system, and all other physiological functions. There is now evidence that deliberate efforts to think certain kinds of thoughts are systematically reflected in changes in regional brain flow and metabolism (Pardo et al. 1991). The only way all these things can happen is for the mental experience to be based upon the brain's apparatus for interacting with the rest of the body. Some have suggested that the mind interacts with the brain without having to obey the laws of thermodynamics (Eccles 1980, Popper and Eccles 1977). To many scientists, this is truly inconceivable and appears to be a way of introducing the concept of the soul into scientific discussions. A less radical view suggests that the mind and brain are inseparable, but acknowledges the current limitations in our understanding of the details concerning the mechanisms for dealing with such concurrence.

Some who argue that the mind and the brain are separable will agree, nevertheless, that medications can affect mood, energy, appetite, sexual drives, sleep, nervousness or anxiety, cognition, learning, memory, etc, and that mental experiences can lead to a wide variety of bodily changes. But they balk when it comes to the *content* of thought, learning, memory, or emotion. And they balk especially when it comes to *intentions*. They resist the belief that neuroscience can ever help us understand the content of our mental experiences. They insist that neuroscience will never be able to help us understand "Shakespeare's insight into psychology," for instance, because such insights are "different in kind from the insights of behavioral psychologists, and both of these [are] different again from the neuroscientific correlates which may be occurring at the same time" (Charlton 1990).

It is certainly the case that we cannot yet provide a credible scientific explanation for the representation in our brains of our thoughts, wishes, fears, goals, ambitions, motives, and all the other varied and rich content of human thinking. *And we may never be able to.* But there is no reason not to be hopeful that we will make important progress.

The evidence linking memory and the brain is so persuasive that few doubt a neural process exists for encoding and storing the verbal or other symbolic content of thought. Over thirty years ago the Canadian neurosurgeon Wilder Penfield (Penfield and Roberts 1959) described what happened when he stimulated electrically highly localized brain areas in conscious patients undergoing surgery for severe, uncontrollable epilepsy. Some patients reported complex and elaborate memories of past experiences closely correlated with the electrical stimulation. These findings strongly suggested that memories are stored in brain cells, which implies some method of coding.

We cannot tell yet what the code for handling language and other such symbols in our brains will be, nor how simple or complex it will prove. Such evaluation can only come after the code is identified. *But it is difficult for many to believe that such a code does not exist.* We think in words or pictures, we hear words and other sounds as music, and we read words and other similar symbols. At the same time, we have no basis for believing that such activities are possible without the brain. And we know that certain brain disturbances adversely affect our ability to carry out such activities. This certainly counts as important evidence in favor of an intimate and inseparable linkage between the brain and the mind.

A remarkably balanced and very clear exposition of the two viewpoints concerning the mind-brain issue was published by A. Rosenberg (1988), a most thoughtful professor of philosophy: "If, as Descartes held, the mind is a substance quite different from the rest of nature, operating in accordance with different principles, then we have the beginnings of an explanation of why its study, psychology, and the study of the consequences of human thoughts and actions, the rest of social science, cannot proceed in the way the study of matter does. Metaphysical differences dictate scientific differences. Descartes argued that the mind was distinct from the body on the grounds that the former has properties no chunk of matter could possibly have. His most famous argument was that our minds have the property of our not being able to doubt their existence, whereas no part of our bodies, including our brains, have this feature."

On the other side of the argument, Rosenberg writes: "Dualism has the greatest difficulty with the evident fact that our mental states have both physical causes and physical effects. It is hard to see how something nonphysical can have such relations. For causation is preeminently a physical relation, one that involves pushes and pulls and the transfer of kinetic energy, which is a function of mass and velocity. But the interpretationalist [one who denies the possibility of explaining at least the content of mental activities in natural science terms] can turn this mystery to advantage. For the impossibility of causal relations between mind and matter provides an explanation of why a predictive science of human behavior, modelled on natural science, is quite impossible." Shifting again, Rosenberg observes the "naturalist has the same problem in reverse, for naturalism purports to absorb the mind to nature and so to explain the appropriateness of methods drawn from the natural sciences to its study. And . . . this is no easy matter. We have as yet no plausible explanation for the most basic fact naturalism rests on: how physical matter can have intentional content, how an arrangement of matter—the brain—can represent other arrangements of physical matter. Yet if the mind is the brain, this is what our beliefs and desires will be."

Some of us do believe that it is possible for an arrangement of matter to represent other arrangements of physical matter. That is just what a book, a film, an audio tape, a computer memory do. Many of us believe that the brain does the same thing—we just do not yet understand the mechanisms for doing it and we do not know the code. When it comes to intentionality we face greater difficulty, because those who believe the brain is the organ of the mind are still stymied by the lack of a satisfactory neural model for intentionality.

These arguments probably will not persuade those who see an unbridgeable gap between mind and brain. The debate is too deep-seated to be resolved until our knowledge of brain function is much greater. We are thus left with two apparently irreconcilable views that have very different implications for the relationship between psychiatry and medical training. The dualist can reject the relevance of medical training. The naturalist, or believer in the mind-brain union, must emphasize the need for medical training.

Psychiatrists who favor the dualist position face several dilemmas. Despite their own medical training, they are without a satisfactory intellectual basis for arguing in favor of medical training for psychiatrists. They have no basis for insisting on the special privileges and opportunities that accrue to them because of their medical training and for resisting the pressures from other mental health professionals to be allowed to exercise the same professional options. Perhaps the most plausible argument they can offer is that since the situation is unsettled the status quo should be maintained.

It seems evident to me that the problems associated with rejecting the dualistic formulation are less severe than those that accompany its acceptance. The former problems can be worked on by research that builds upon past successes. The latter problems seem to offer no hope of solution.

Reductionism

Reductionism is an issue that invariably arises in discussions of mind-brain relationships. The general issue is whether phenomena at one level of description can be explained at another more "basic" level, for example, chemical reactions in terms of principles of physics, biological processes in terms of chemical reactions, or sociological observations in terms of psychological processes. In biological psychiatry the debate is often whether it is appropriate to try to explain at least certain psychological experiences (thoughts, intentions, wishes, goals) in terms of cellular and molecular processes.

Traditionally, this debate has been framed in terms of two extreme and incompatible positions. One view is that ultimately it should be possible to "explain" descriptions at the level of subjective experience concerning feelings, thoughts, intentions, and so on in terms of descriptions at the level of physiology or molecular and cellular processes. The other is that it will never be possible to describe human subjective experiences in such terms.

If reductionism is construed in absolute terms, any useful resolution of the debate appears unlikely. If reductionist explanations are required to be total, there is little possibility that they can ever be completely successful. For example, if a reductionistic approach demands that neurophysiology be able to explain everything about one's subjective emotional and intellectual experience on listening to Beethoven's ninth symphony, few would be so bold as to assert that this will be possible in the foreseeable future. On the other hand, if reductionism is conceptualized as involving different levels of success, there appears to be merit in applying it as far as one is able.

There are very few, if any, complete reductionist explanations for most chemical reactions or for most physiological processes (Churchland and Churchland 1990), much less psychological ones. Despite this, chemists and physiologists do not categorically reject reductionist explanations when they seem to work, just because they cannot account for many other phenomena in the same way. Most if not all reductionist explanations in biology are partial, but nonetheless useful. Science could hardly progress without them.

Only rarely in science is it feasible to completely substitute explanations at a "basic" level of description for a less basic one. Chemists usually cannot abandon chemical descriptions and go directly to explanations in terms of physics. And physiologists still need to use physiological rather than chemical descriptions. In all fields of medicine, it is usually impossible to avoid clinical levels of description and analysis.

Free Will

This age-old issue confronts us with what appear to be two incompatible viewpoints. On one hand, everyone is subjectively convinced of his or her capacity to make choices, initiate actions, and resist all sorts of pressures from outside and from within. On the other, we are clearly subject to conditions, both genetic and environmental that shape if not entirely determine our behavior. If we do not have free will, we cannot be conceived of as responsible individuals; there can be no valid morality.

Very few psychiatrists ignore the possibility, and even probability, that many of our patients' thoughts, emotions, and overt behaviors are determined, at least in part, by processes over which they have limited if any control. Most of us believe that this is the case when patients experience delusions, hallucinations, mania, depression, obsessions, compulsions, panic attacks, phobias, habituations and addictions to various substances, atypical sexual orientations, and so on. This contributes to our view that these experiences constitute illness.

At the same time, most of us also believe that some patients, especially with professional help, can partially control some of these experiences. All forms of psychotherapy assume that with help some patients can modify their behavior, thinking, or emotional responses. In short, we seem to hold contradictory ideas. We often show the same apparent contradictions when it comes to patients' responsibility for their behavior. We may be prepared to argue that some patients should not be held responsible for their behavior (e.g., psychotic individuals) but that others should be (e.g., those with antisocial personality).

It seems most reasonable to me to adopt the view that questions about free will are best answered empirically, rather than by reasoning from certain axioms. This means we ought to be open-minded in the absence of convincing evidence. Unlike philosophers, psychiatrists often have to deal with the question of free will case by case. We know that it is possible to predict some behaviors, within specifiable statistical limits of confidence. This means of course that some of our behavior is strongly conditioned by physiological or social factors, even though people often are not fully aware of the impact of these factors. Simultaneously, we know that much human behavior is not predictable. This does not mean it is entirely unconditioned but implies that the links are looser or that other factors may also be operating. ᵢₙₒᵤ complexly determined

For some at least, among such other factors may be free will. This means that changes must be expected in the *manifest* scope of free will as antecedents of choice and behavior are studied and probed. It seems likely that much of our choice is constrained to some degree. In some areas, the constraint will be modest; in other areas, great. It also seems likely that individuals will vary on these attributes just as they do on most others. Viewed this way, questions concerning free will should lose their power to force us into seemingly contradictory and incompatible positions when we try to understand the nature of psychiatric disorders and our efforts to treat them.

For example, most clinicians believe that psychotic patients have little or no control over their hallucinations and delusions. Yet, they also believe that it is sometimes possible to help patients alter their responses to such psychotic experiences. Some psychotic patients commit crimes under the influence of their psychotic ideation after resisting for long periods of time, and knowing that what they do is wrong. At the same time, other patients seem able to resist indefinitely.

Anglo-Saxon legal theory traditionally assigns guilt only if the perpetrator of the crime is of "sound mind." The meaning of this criterion and its relationship to free will have been the basis for much debate within legal and psychiatric circles. The concept of "sound mind" is still not applied consistently, probably because of limitations in psychiatric knowledge.

When psychiatrists enter the courtroom, they usually cannot estimate the degree to which patients can exercise their free will. It usually seems reasonable to conclude that, with regard to their symptoms and behavior, patients have varying degrees of control or choice. Another way to put it is that "patients have free will, but not equally about everything and at all times."

A thoughtful book by the philosopher Daniel C. Dennett helps clarify the question of free will. He sets the stage by reminding us early that "Ideas about causation were at the focus of attention in the early days of Greek philosophy, and it occurred to some to wonder whether all physical events are caused or determined by the sum total of all prior events. If they are—if, as we say, *determinism* is true—then our actions, as physical events, must themselves be determined. If determinism is true, then our every deed and decision is the inexorable outcome, it seems, of the sum of physical forces acting at the moment, which in turn is the inexorable outcome of the forces acting an instant before, and so on, to the beginning of time." This leads to the question: "How then could we be free?"

Referring to his earlier interest in sculpting as a career, he proposes the use of the tactics of the sculptor to deal with philosophical issues, including free will. "Unlike the draftsman, who must get each line right with the first stroke of the pen, the sculptor has the luxury of nibbling and grinding away until the lines and surfaces look just right. First you rough out the block, standing back and squinting now and then to make sure you are closing in on the dimly seen final product. Only after the piece is bulked out in the right proportions do you return to each crude, rough surface and invest great labor in getting the fine details just so."

This is an elegant way of expressing what was proposed above. We may not be able to deal with all the questions concerning free will in one fell swoop. It may require working on pieces of the argument until we have learned enough to provide the complete "clear, well-supported, soundly reasoned answers."

Dennett argues that there are many unknowns and unknowables when we try to understand what free will might and might not signify. To return to his metaphor of the sculptor, we may not yet be ready to work on the "fine details," and, in fact, may still be very vague about the "final product." It may even turn out that the final product will be quite different from what we think we are after.

To restate the arguments: in an agnostic way, we must be ready to categorize as free will whatever behavior we are unable to predict and that the individual believes to be the result of his or her intent. To paraphrase Dennett, very few of us can choose to do many things we might like to do, either because of external sanctions or because of our own limitations. Many also appreciate that our choices are conditioned by many forces we may be only dimly aware of or of which we are entirely unconscious. We should try to understand the constraints on free will through empirical research rather than by logical reasoning from assumptions or axioms that may not be valid. Inevitably, we will be forced to accept uncertainty and ambiguity in many cases.

Consciousness

Consciousness is something we are all aware of and yet it is not easy to define precisely. Whatever else it may mean, however, consciousness involves subjective awareness of our environment and of our mental experiences. For many, it is a most characteristically human trait. It is tightly linked to our capacity to be introspective, consider the implications of experiences, and weigh decisions. Since Descartes, if not before, it has been the foundation of our belief in reality: "Cogito, ergo sum," since I am aware and able to think, I know that I exist. In this discussion I will assume that consciousness is a special characteristic of humans, that there are less developed forms of it in some other animals, and that it is linked inseparably to the brain.

Psychiatrists are inevitably concerned with the matter of consciousness. Most of our time with patients is spent trying to understand their conscious experiences, including their symptoms. We also face questions about nonconscious processes. Often our patients have experiences that they cannot explain at all or only inadequately, such as hallucinations, delusions, obsessions, compulsions, phobias, or panic attacks. In addition, patients often cannot account for their disturbances in mood and affect, such as depression, mania, and anxiety. This question of non-conscious reasons for our experiences is really at the heart of psychiatric interest in consciousness. We are all interested in the possibility that conscious mental processes and experiences can be affected by processes and experiences of which we are not aware.

There appear to be at least two main kinds of non-conscious processes. One kind presumably shares many of the same characteristics seen in conscious process in that the non-conscious experience has once been conscious or can become so under appropriate circumstances, but is somehow prevented from becoming conscious by various controlling or modifying processes. The out-of-awareness state of a memory may be the result of some failure in the brain's scanning and retrieval system or of some normal inhibitory system, perhaps evolved to permit the organism to concentrate on immediate problems without inappropriate distraction, or of some normal or even abnormal system of attenuation or loss of the database of coded experiences.

The second kind of non-conscious process differs from the first in that it was never conscious and cannot be made conscious in any significant way. Here, I am referring to the many bodily processes, including brain processes, which are entirely, or nearly entirely, beyond our capacity to recognize consciously but which nevertheless can and do profoundly influence our conscious thinking and feeling. These brain and other bodily mechanisms involve the many biochemical and physiological systems that interact with those subserving consciousness and hence mental experiences.

Thus far, most psychiatrists probably can more or less agree. The main divergence is encountered in the psychoanalytic concept of the "dynamic unconscious," referring to the putative non-conscious processes that either were conscious at one time or can be made conscious through the interpretation of symptoms, dreams, slips of the tongue, and, most important, free associations. According to the psychoanalytic view, the non-conscious mental content is kept that way through the action of unconscious defense mechanisms, especially repression. The psychoanalytic view puts major emphasis on unconscious conflicts as central to the etiology of psychiatric disorders.

Freudian teaching and practice have traditionally emphasized the hypotheses that it is particularly *certain* unconscious processes, *those that are similar to conscious processes in that they are capable of being made conscious*, that are the key to understanding psychopathology. This hypothesis may be historically understandable, but it seems no longer satisfactory or reasonable to limit the concept of non-conscious to those processes that were or can be made conscious. As argued in Chapter 4, it appears highly probable that non-conscious processes, which never can become accessible to the techniques of psychoanalysis or other forms of psychotherapeutic exploration, are causally related to many psychiatric conditions.

Recent research concerning lateralization of brain functions has opened new ways of thinking and studying consciousness (Gazzaniga 1985, Geschwind and Galaburda 1987, Gruzelier and Flor-Henry 1979). Studies of brain lateralization were greatly stimulated by fascinating work with so-called split-brain cases, individuals who have had the corpus callosum severed surgically so as to reduce the propagation of aberrant electrical activity leading to severe and intractable grand mal seizures (Gazzaniga 1985). This research has made it clear that there are consistent patterns in the differentiation of functions between the two brain hemispheres. But of great significance for consciousness is the evidence that when the connections between the two hemispheres are extensively, if not wholly, severed, each of the two hemispheres appears to have different mental experiences of which the opposite hemisphere seems to be unaware!

Of interest to psychiatrists are hypotheses that some forms of psychopathology, including hallucinations and their elaborations into delusional explanations, may result from impairment of the normal suppression of the non-dominant hemisphere by the dominant hemisphere (Crow et al. 1989, Early 1990, 1991, Pardo et al. 1991). These hypotheses raise the possibility that some cases of schizophrenia, for example, may reflect subtle alterations in the normal processes of brain lateralization. It is at least conceivable that some hallucinations arise from the non-dominant hemisphere when the dominant hemisphere's suppressive functions are impaired.

A few brief quotations from Gazzaniga, a pioneer and leader in this area of research, may be helpful in considering such hypotheses. "One of the most compelling features of split-brain surgery is the fact that the patient's behavior, affect, and general personality are totally untouched. Having the left brain disconnected from the right does not produce disturbances in everyday life, and the untrained eye would find it difficult to detail that a patient had surgery at all. The dramatic effects can be observed only under careful laboratory conditions using the same procedures as our preoperative testing (Gazzaniga 1985, page 41). . . . The upshot of these first efforts was that the animal work was confirmed in man—the cutting of the cerebral commisures produced two separate mental systems, each with its own capacity to learn, remember, feel emotion, and behave. The notion that man is an indivisible agent becomes questionable (page 44)." He explicitly goes on to propose that each of the divided hemispheres has its own separate consciousness.

One of Gazzaniga's concepts may even add a third category to the kinds of non-conscious experiences described above: "coconscious but nonverbal mental modules," referring to some of the functions of the non-dominant hemisphere, usually the right, following surgical division of the corpus callosum. This suggests a form of awareness that cannot be verbalized in the absence of an intact connection to the dominant hemisphere with its capacity for language. He argues that these modules have "a response tendency, a decision for action . . . [that] is not unconscious. It is very conscious, very capable of effecting action."

These investigations make clear that even consciousness, that central but elusive concept of philosophy, can be studied scientifically and that investigation into the details of the brain's structure and function can contribute dramatically to our better understanding of philosophical questions as well as of psychiatric conditions.

The Meaning of Illness

Many people try to fit the experience of illness into their framework for justifying or rationalizing all experience in philosophical, religious, or other transcendental terms.

For some individuals, the process is relatively straightforward. Their faith in God provides the basis for assigning significance to everything that happens, including illness, pain, suffering, and death. God has purposes that we are not privileged to know and understand, and our task is to accept what He prescribes for us, confident that, in time, it will turn out for the best. For many others in modern society, such faith is not easy to attain, but they may rely on other philosophical or personal beliefs to rationalize their experiences.

Experienced physicians of all kinds are not surprised at the frequency with which patients and their families make comments or ask questions that reflect the concern: Why is this happening to me (or him or her)? Because psychiatric disorders are more difficult for patients and relatives to conceptualize, psychiatrists encounter this question in one form or another frequently. Because psychiatric illnesses are manifested primarily as alterations in the way a person reacts to life's experiences, and because patients and their families are prone to interpret such conditions in terms of meaningful psychosocial experiences, they often wonder about the significance of the illness.

For example, patients suffering from depression, which is frequently accompanied by strong guilt feelings, may torment themselves over past sins for which they are now being punished. Similarly, patients with schizophrenia, who tend to misinterpret the world and people around them, commonly conclude that they are victims of a conspiracy on the part of some church, political organization, or other organized group. Patients suffering from mania sometimes also interpret their altered thinking and behavior to mean that God has a special mission for them.

Another reason why questions about the significance of illness are common in psychiatric practice relates to psychodynamic approaches to psychiatry, which have become part of the conventional wisdom in so much of our society. Because of the main assumption underlying such psychodynamic ideas—that the understanding of behavior in general and of psychiatric illness in particular is to be found in our unconscious minds and that through treatment what is unconscious can be made conscious—it is not surprising that many patients want to discuss the meaning of their illnesses.

But there is another basis for interest in the meaning of illness that derives from the efforts of philosophers to understand the nature of knowing. This field is referred to as epistemology. It is especially concerned with what constitutes valid evidence and how we are to make judgments about conflicting claims to knowledge that arise from different conceptual and methodologic strategies. The major difference here is between those who are committed to natural science strategies and those who deny that this is the only or even the best approach to understanding human behavior.

The argument put forward by adherents of this latter view is that human behavior stems from complex historical, social, and psychological forces that cannot be rationalized or understood by means of a deterministic, natural science theory of causality. The goal of research, according to this view, is to make human experience "more intelligible" rather than "more predictable," which is the way Rosenberg (1988) epitomizes the differences in approach between the two philosophical camps. Behavior can be made intelligible if it is given "meaning" characterized by a plausible story that is itself founded on religious, cultural, philosophical, or other beliefs.

Rosenberg insists that it is not truly possible to avoid making a choice between these two very different approaches to knowledge. He also argues that it is not reasonable to "accept a permanent agnosticism about the claims of incompatible theories of knowledge." Some may prefer to remain agnostic, however. This must present them with many dilemmas and serious contradictions. Others may be prepared to maintain that "understanding" or "meaning" rather than "prediction" is what we must accept for psychological or social phenomena. My view is that "understanding" as knowledge, in contrast to "prediction" or "control" as knowledge, is not compatible with science, as it is generally understood, at least in biomedical research. Certainly, an approach to knowledge concerning psychiatric conditions that is based on an epistemology of "understanding" removes it from the domain of science as it is conceived in medicine.

This very important distinction between two philosophical positions may help illuminate some of the problems psychiatry faces as it tries to define its place in relation to the rest of medicine. Few physicians outside of psychiatry are prepared to accept "meaning" or "understanding" in this context as properly within the field of medical science. To the degree that they confront psychiatrists advocating this epistemological view, a serious gap develops even when the other physicians find the proposed meaning interesting and even reasonable.

The attribution of meaning within the polarization described by Rosenberg may reflect a basic characteristic of the human mind, but the validation of any particular meaning outside of the strategies of natural science does not appear to be possible within the traditions and practices of natural science. In the care of patients and in dealing with their relatives and friends, physicians, including psychiatrists, may have to accept and deal with meanings patients assign to their experience of illness. But it remains necessary to distinguish between what may be scientifically validated and what lies outside the realm of scientific explanation, even if for some it appears to reflect an inescapable need.

It may not be possible for psychiatrists or others to achieve consensus about the meaning of illness. But all of us need to understand the implications of whichever of the two sides in the debate we choose. The medical model makes it very difficult, probably impossible, to accept the meaning of illness as a substitute for knowledge concerning etiology and pathogenesis.

Ethics

Psychiatry shares most of the ethical concerns that permeate the rest of medicine, but some are particularly important in psychiatry because of the nature of psychiatric illness. The central ethical issue that is characteristically psychiatric has to do with the obligations and responsibilities psychiatrists face in dealing with patients whose illnesses interfere with their judgment and create threats to themselves as well as to others. This clearly has a legal dimension that sometimes complicates decisions and sometimes makes them easier.

No other ethical issue that psychiatrists face as physicians touches on their views about the nature of psychiatric illness so much as the patient's potential for harm to self or others. Psychiatrists who deny the validity of the medical model are likely to reach very different conclusions concerning professional responsibility than those who accept the model with its many implications.

No one has articulated the anti-medical position more strongly and consistently than Thomas Szasz, a psychiatrist and psychoanalyst of considerable renown. In a long series of books, articles, and lectures, he has vehemently and relentlessly argued that mental illness is a "myth" (Szasz 1961) and that involuntary psychiatric hospitalization resembles "the Oriental despotic arbitrariness towards troublesome persons much more closely than the Occidental legal respect towards persons accused of crimes (Szasz 1989). His arguments have not been motivated simply by a desire to minimize the risk of errors in judgment and practice by psychiatrists or lawyers—errors that have led to mistreatment of psychiatric patients. Rather, he has been trying to undermine the very idea of mental illness as a valid concept. He recognizes no basis for a medical approach to what are called psychiatric conditions and accepts no justification for involuntary psychiatric hospitalization.

Szasz claims that *all* psychiatric disorders are "metaphors," that calling people "sick" who suffer from a psychiatric condition is the same as referring to a "sick" economy or a "sick" world. It is his position that there are "two diametrically opposed points of view about mental illness and psychiatry. According to the traditional and at present generally accepted view, mental illness is like any other illness; psychiatric treatment is like any other treatment; and psychiatry is like any other specialty. According to the view I have endeavored to develop and clarify, however, there is, and can be, no such thing as mental illness or psychiatric treatment; the interventions now designated as 'psychiatric treatment' must be clearly identified as voluntary or involuntary: voluntary interventions are things a person does for himself in an effort to change, whereas involuntary interventions are things done to him in an effort to change him against his will; and psychiatry is not a medical but a moral and political enterprise" (Szasz 1973).

Szasz has been consistent in his arguments. He has even written about the "myth of psychotherapy. . . . Psychotherapeutic interventions are metaphorical treatments that stand in the same sort of relation to medical treatments as criticizing and editing television programs stand to repairing television receivers. Simply put, psychotherapy is conversation, and conversation is not treatment. All forms of psychotherapy rest on and constitute the practice of some sort of ethic, usually of a secular sort" (Szasz 1974).

Szasz began writing and talking this way about thirty years ago. This was early in the development of modern psychopharmacology and before the great expansion of research into the genetic and neurobiological components of psychiatric disorders. Nevertheless, he is quoted extensively here because he has never retracted or modified any of his important arguments and because his ideas have influenced many people, especially outside the medical profession. In earlier sections of this book, the problems with his viewpoint were discussed (see chapters 1 and 4) and there is little need to repeat. Szasz's position, though, sets the stage for a discussion of the central ethical questions in psychiatry.

The possibility of involuntary psychiatric hospitalization is usually considered when an individual is believed to be suffering from a psychiatric disorder and is manifesting strong suicidal tendencies or strong homicidal and other violent tendencies, or shows significant impairment in the capacity to care for himself without help and is refusing all such help. Involuntary hospitalization is resorted to when such an individual cannot be persuaded to enter the hospital voluntarily for treatment of the psychiatric disorder.

Szasz would argue that an individual with a history of recurrent depression and mania, who had made a previous, medically serious suicide attempt, and is now thinking about shooting himself, should never be hospitalized against his will because we do not yet have any evidence that the recurrent mood disturbances are the result of some brain pathology (his only criterion for accepting a psychiatric disorder as a medical condition). Further, he would say that this individual has the right, as everyone does, to commit suicide without hindrance. He recognizes no valid distinction between an individual with a history of psychiatric difficulties and one who does not have such a history. He even claims that the psychiatrist has no professional responsbility to try to prevent suicide (Szasz 1971).

Szasz apparently does not attach any importance to the many studies of suicides clearly demonstrating that suicide usually is committed by persons with a severe or prolonged psychiatric illness and does not occur randomly. Major affective disorder, schizophrenia, alcoholism, and other substance abuse are present in the great majority of cases, based upon systematic "psychological autopsies" of consecutive cases of suicide (see Robins 1981 for references).

Szasz truly is an example of his point that: "In language and logic we are the prisoners of our premises, just as in politics and law we are the prisoners of our rulers. Hence we had better pick them well."

If one believes that depression, mania, schizophrenia, and other psychiatric conditions are not illnesses, one has no ethical dilemma. If one sees no reason ever to hospitalize individuals with such conditions against their will, one has no ethical dilemma. If one rejects any professional responsibility to prevent suicide or physical harm to others by any individual, one has no ethical dilemma. It would follow that one should feel no misgiving if one's patient or client committed suicide or seriously injured another while under one's care.

On the other hand, psychiatrists who accept the medical model and take the studies of suicide seriously must confront the ethical dilemma of deciding whether to force patients into the hospital and into certain treatments. We can contemplate such actions when we believe our patients are suffering from illnesses that are adversely affecting their insight and judgment and that may lead to great harm. At the same time, we must be alert to errors in professional judgment, and we should welcome review through the procedures of our legal system.

It is certainly true that involuntary hospitalization at times has been initiated and continued without enough attention to what is professionally valid and legally permissible. Many such cases have provoked legal challenges that have led to great improvements in the way these dilemmas are now approached. But we must continue to be alert to any risk of abuse and take great care to use involuntary hospitalization only when there is a reasonable basis to fear that a patient's behavior, *because of the nature of the underlying psychiatric disorder*, may result in material harm to self or others. We must also be sure that those charged with the patient's care are required to have their evaluation of the patient and the patient's progress reviewed promptly and frequently, again through established judicial process. We should expect to meet more stringent criteria for continuing involuntary hospitalization than for initiating it.

Involuntary hospitalization is permitted under our laws only when the patient's illness is such that the patient's thinking, judgment, and self-control are significantly impaired, the patient is seriously contemplating action that constitutes a serious threat to self or others, and the patient refuses to cooperate with treatment. Often only a very brief period of hospitalization is necessary to bring about sufficient improvement in the patient's illness to permit continued treatment under voluntary conditions. Occasionally, a few days of involuntary hospitalization make it clear that the risks associated with the patient's disorder are less than seemed to be the case at first, thus also permitting release from any legal constraints on the patient's freedom. Finally, in some clinical circumstances, further observation confirms the need for continued treatment on an involuntary basis because the patient is still showing the same clinical features that led to involuntary hospitalization and remains unwilling to cooperate in treatment. Frequent judicial review is called for under these circumstances. The aim is to continue involuntary hospitalization for the shortest time possible, consistent with the patient's clinical condition.

The last admonition carries with it certain implications that the patient, the patient's relatives and friends, and the larger public must understand. The psychiatrist's ability to make judgments about the kinds of risks that lead to involuntary hospitalization and treatment is limited and errors in judgment are inevitable. A society that values personal freedom as strongly as ours must constantly weigh the costs and benefits of alternative strategies. The price to be paid for striving to avoid mistakes by easy and prolonged involuntary hospitalization can mean serious erosion of constitutional rights. The price for taking the opposite tack is that more people may commit suicide or be killed or injured by psychiatrically ill individuals. We cannot avoid struggling with these dilemmas.

Some people may be more comfortable with constraints on patients who threaten violence to others than on patients who seem to constitute threats only to themselves. They might argue that we should not use involuntary hospitalization and treatment to try to prevent suicide or serious suicide attempts. Fundamental to this position is the principle that individuals may be constrained, at least under certain very limited circumstances, when it comes to injuring others but not when they are injuring only themselves. I am very sympathetic to this principle in general, but, as one who believes in the validity of psychiatric illness, I must accept the need to modify the application of the principle to a certain degree in the presence of certain clinical conditions.

Research findings are very consistent around the world: the great majority of individuals who commit suicide and many who only make suicide attempts are suffering from depression or another serious psychiatric disorder. Many of those who commit suicide have seen physicians within a few months of the suicide, with complaints and symptoms that, in retrospect at least, indicate they were suffering from a recognizable psychiatric illness at the time. Comparatively few individuals commit suicide because they are suffering from a painful, disabling, life-threatening general medical illness, such as cancer or cardiovascular disease, which together account for nearly three-quarters of all deaths in the United States. And finally, very few individuals in our society commit suicide because they are expressing some cultural or social imperative, such as a response to disgrace.

In the face of such data, the psychiatrist who is persuaded that psychiatric disorders are best viewed as illnesses comparable to epilepsy, cardiac arrhythmias, or even coronary artery atherosclerosis, is under great pressure to try to treat patients with such psychiatric disorders. Further, knowing that suicide is an all too frequent complication of many psychiatric conditions, it seems reasonable to try to prevent or at least postpone suicide while trying to treat the underlying psychiatric illness.

Though all this supports the argument for an aggressive effort to prevent suicide, there are situations where I stop making this effort. Many of us have seen patients with profoundly disabling psychiatric conditions that have proven largely resistant to treatment. Sometimes, such patients insist that they can no longer sustain the suffering. They argue that, having tried many different interventions without success and continuing to experience pain and misery over many years, they have a right to consider suicide.

In my own clinical experience, there have been a few cases where I have agreed with the patient and accepted the need to forego any effort to force him or her into the hospital to prevent suicide. I have not done so, however, until I have been satisfied that the patient has tried all reasonable treatments and continues to suffer very severely. Needless to say, I believe strongly that this decision should be made only after considerable discussion with the patient and family.

My position in such cases is not different from what it is when confronted by the occasional patient suffering from metastatic cancer or some other painful and severely disabling general medical condition who seriously seems to be contemplating suicide. In such cases, I would not rigidly insist on protecting the patient from his or her intentions. Instead I see my responsibility as trying to engage the patient, and the patient's family, in what are I hope psychotherapeutic discussions about all aspects of the patient's situation and options.

I can understand a colleague whose views rule out any lessening of therapeutic efforts, right up to the end of the patient's life, in this clinical situation. I might disagree with his or her ethical assumptions, but I can be sympathetic if the physician has clearly informed the patient and the patient's family about his or her ethical position and has offered to turn over the patient's care to a physician with different ethical assumptions. I have more difficulty accepting a position like Szasz's unless the patient and family have been clearly informed that there is no intention to treat the patient's condition as an illness and, therefore, that the therapist is not prepared to accept the responsibilities normally associated with a doctor-patient relationship including the obligation to try to prevent suicide and treat the underlying illness in conformity with the limitations discussed above.

Where I do agree with Szasz is that our assumptions about psychiatry are of profound importance. They greatly shape our expectations, our ethical positions, and our approach to treatment. Arguing for the medical model is more than an abstract intellectual debate; it has many practical implications.

7

Education, Training, and Research

These terms cover the academic aspects of psychiatry. In medicine, generally, education refers to the study of the principles and elements of medicine, including its various specialties, such as psychiatry, and the relevant basic sciences. The term is commonly applied to the four years of medical school. Training, on the other hand, refers to learning how the concepts and principles are applied to the actual care of individual patients. The term is typically used to describe what takes place during a residency or other post-residency program. There is considerable overlap between medical education and training, which actually represent an indivisible continuum. Research is often coupled with education and training because of the strong conviction among many teachers of all branches of medicine, which the author shares, that, on average, the best education and training in medicine are to be had in an environment that fosters research.

Education and Training and the Medical Model

The argument presented here reflects the belief that the education and training of medical students and residents in psychiatry are best shaped by the medical model. At the same time, however, they need to include an understanding of other major perspectives or models and of the major philosophical issues concerning psychiatry encountered during clinical experiences.

Students and residents need opportunities to study and work with a wide variety of patients so as to extend and improve their clinical skills of interviewing and assessing patients and applying common treatments. They need to observe and practice carrying out mental status examinations. They must consider the findings of their own and other examinations to clarify the meaning of the many elements of the psychiatric examination and appreciate the variations to be seen in each one. They need to practice interviewing different kinds of patients from different backgrounds and under different circumstances. This should include patients in the emergency room, psychiatric inpatient service, psychiatric outpatient clinic, and patients seen in consultation on the medical and surgical services of the general hospital.

Students and residents must learn how important it is to talk to relatives and friends about the patient's troubles as well as to establish the kind of relationship with the family that will support the treatment program. They need to discover that there is no such thing as a complete history. They have to understand that eliciting the patient's history is an evolving process, which can be facilitated by ongoing efforts to clarify and elaborate the various elements of the history as the relationship between the patient and physician develops. New information, from the patient, relatives, nurses, and the results of different diagnostic studies, should trigger additional efforts to be sure that one understands the patient's experiences and history and that the patient understands the physician's questions and comments.

Students and residents need to learn and appreciate that the history of the patient's medical experiences elicited from the patient and relatives will be affected by many factors. It is to be expected that everyone's understanding of questions and memory of events will be modified, to varying degrees of course, by concerns and fears about illness, treatment, disability, and death. Psychiatric illness is, in addition, often accompanied by guilt, feelings of self-deprecation, suspiciousness, cognitive impairment, and often profound demoralization and pessimism. Obviously, these will also affect the history obtained. Eliciting the most accurate and objective history possible is the goal; patience, time, and interest from the physician are essential if the goal is to be achieved.

Students and trainees need supervised experience in the use of various psychotherapeutic techniques, psychopharmacologic agents, behavior modification, ECT, and other interventions, in relationship to their educational level. They must learn how to work effectively with physicians in other specialties and with other mental health professionals. They need to develop familiarity with the application of laboratory studies to the evaluation of their patients, including new brain-imaging technologies. They need to develop reasonable sophistication about the use of various psychological tests; this should include some understanding of the theories behind the tests and a grasp of the way different test results have been validated.

To varying degrees, depending on the subject, students and residents must become familiar with the original literature in psychiatry. They must have opportunities to review selected papers critically for the purpose of carefully thinking out the way a question or problem was formulated and approached. They need to consider the methods used—for selecting subjects or materials, for choosing controls, for measurement or other description, for analyzing the results, and for drawing conclusions. The spirit of such critique should be to make it clear how hard it is to answer certain questions and how difficult it can be to be sure about the validity of the answers. A regular challenge should be to consider how the study might have been better designed and executed. Such review of published work provides an excellent vehicle to strengthen the educational experience. Such critical reading and discussion offer the best process for nailing down one's knowledge and estimating the confidence one ought to place on that knowledge. Students and residents need to be helped to acquire the self-confidence that comes from thoughtful study of any subject, so that they will feel able to review someone's work and ideas and discuss the subject with their peers in a constructive and critical fashion.

Teachers as Role Models

To these ends, students and residents need teachers who will serve as good role models. Such teachers need to be comfortable with the goals specified above. They should have little need to appear omniscient or infallible. They ought to be comfortable in acknowledging ignorance or uncertainty and open to suggestions and challenges from those they are teaching. They should be very clear in their teaching concerning the differences between what is conventional wisdom and what is based on valid data. They should be temperamentally predisposed to encouraging a truly questioning approach from their students and residents.

All experienced clinical teachers have their own favorite questions to pose to those they are teaching. Some of my favorites are useful for starting discussions about all sorts of issues in psychiatry. Is this patient sick? What do you mean by sickness here? How would you respond to someone who challenged you with Dr. Szasz's dictum that mental illness is a myth? What does it mean to you that I elicited a different story from the one you got? What might it mean that we can achieve a greater consensus that the patient is thinking about suicide than that the patient is showing a blunted affect? What ideas do you have about the significance of diurnal variation? Do you know why the patient came into the hospital (or emergency room or clinic) yesterday rather than last week? Might it be a good sign that the patient is not fully compliant?

Such questions are not meant to elicit some "correct" answer. The purpose is to stimulate thinking and discussion about the many possible ways of approaching clinical problems in psychiatry, which can open up related issues as well. The discussions can provide opportunities to suggest reading that can lead to further consideration of the issues. The aim should always be to include conceptual and attitudinal concerns as well as more factual ones.

Discussions of a report in the literature can be facilitated by certain questions. Is the author clear about the question he or she set out to answer? Is it clear how the author selected the sample and controls? Was this the best sample for the question? What potential biases seem possible given the study design? Could these have been avoided? How do they affect the results and conclusions? Are the author's findings consistent with those of others studying similar questions? If not, what might explain the different results? Can you suggest a way to clarify the different results through a new study or additional analysis of the data? What are possible implications for clinical practice of this report?

Regardless of the particular question or comment, we must repeatedly remind students and residents to accept responsibility for their continuing education. While their teachers can provide role models and structured learning situations like rounds, conferences, seminars, and supervised care of patients, the students and residents must appreciate the importance of their own ongoing, self-directed efforts. One question I like to ask a medical student who has just presented a case on rounds is, "What did you learn from studying this patient that you did not know before?" Students should be concerned about their educational experience if something new and important is not learned from new patients.

Satisfaction in Medical Practice

Critical thinking and self-education in medicine can be fun. They provide the essential elements for enjoying the practice of medicine (Guze 1979), yet it appears that too many physicians fail to achieve such enjoyment consistently over their entire careers. It should be evident to all students, residents, and practicing physicians that the enormous investment in time, money, and commitment typically necessary to become a physician makes no sense if practicing medicine frequently fails to be interesting and enjoyable. Surely there are easier ways to make as much money, if the satisfactions that can be gained in medicine are not forthcoming.

I have written elsewhere (Guze 1979) of four kinds of satisfaction in practicing medicine: prestige, income, helping to relieve suffering, and intellectual stimulation. Prestige and money, as important as they can be, are not sufficient for the long haul. Helping people who are in pain or otherwise suffering is a different matter. Few physicians fail to respond to this satisfaction. And it is just because physicians can often relieve pain and suffering and even postpone untimely death that society has been so generous with its honors and more tangible rewards. If physicians could always relieve pain and other suffering, nothing more would be needed.

Unfortunately, medicine is a long way from such powers and almost certainly will never achieve them. Often enough the physician is able to make only a modest difference. Patients who continue to suffer and complain despite our efforts, whose disorders persist in defying our understanding and knowledge, and who seem perversely unwilling or unable to follow our advice, are the ones who upset and frustrate us, sometimes even anger us. They reinforce our self-doubts and destroy the illusions of omniscience and omnipotence that have always been ready to ensnare the medical profession. We tend to disparage them and their complaints in the way we talk about them. We may blame them for their troubles, and may act as though they do not deserve our professional attention. They fail to meet our expectations as to what a "good patient" is supposed to be like, and we fail to see the very failure in meeting our expectations as an important clinical sign.

Physicians reveal their frustration and dissatisfaction with clinical medicine in several ways. Today there is widespread discouragement among physicians about the mounting restrictions and controls over medical practice that have arisen out of the malpractice crisis and efforts at cost containment. Few of us have not been touched by these developments, and it becomes easier to understand the reasons of those who are ready to retire early and also discourage young people from studying medicine. But there are many reasons to believe the dissatisfaction existed even before the recent changes in the socioeconomic climate in which medicine is practiced. This brings us back to the satisfactions to be had in medicine and, especially, to intellectual stimulation.

After only a few years of practice, some physicians no longer seem to enjoy what they do. They communicate, directly and indirectly, a sense of disappointment, boredom, and even resentment toward medical practice. They very rarely seem to be excited by a challenging case. They disparage the value of continuing education, and are cynical about the value of research for clinical medicine. They reveal no sense of identity with being members of a learned profession. Their professional reading becomes perfunctory, they seldom attend medical meetings, and they give every indication of being in an intellectual rut.

One cannot avoid asking, how does this happen? What keeps physicians from being engaged by the intellectual challenge of medicine? Undoubtedly, many important factors contribute to this unhappy condition, but it is hard to avoid concluding that their education and training were defective in important ways.

To achieve the goal of continued intellectual stimulation from practice, the physician, beginning in medical school, must cultivate an approach to medicine that is questioning, critical, and curious. Each patient can be viewed as offering a genuine chance to learn something and to test one's experiences against those of others as reflected in textbooks and journal articles. Medical practice can be conceived as an opportunity for clinical research. This can open up all sorts of stimulating and even important questions to study, which can then contribute to the satisfactions of practice.

Too often, students and residents have had very little encouragement or opportunity to become interested in all aspects of their patients' problems. Their concept of working with patients does not include the idea that the way the patient approaches the doctor, describes the presenting complaints, responds to the physician's questions and comments, reacts to the illness and the treatment, fails to cooperate, or tries to manipulate the doctor and the system, are all clinical manifestations that the physician can approach in exctly the same way that the physician approaches a rash, hemorrhages in the eyegrounds, a diastolic murmur, blood in the urine, and so on. In all these latter situations, the physician is trained to think about differential diagnostic possibilities, possible therapeutic interventions, pathogenetic processes, prognostic implications, and so on. Similar reactions are possible when it comes to the salient behavioral features evident in the particular patient. Diagnostic, therapeutic, epidemiologic, and pathogenetic possibilities should be considered here as well, and the relevant literature also reviewed as appropriate. Most important, the physician builds up a database of personal experience that helps shape future practice and sometimes provides an opportunity to contribute to the literature.

In other words, too many physicians approach patients with a narrow concept as to what is properly of clinical concern. Everything outside this narrow concept is therefore regarded as a distraction, to be regretted politely at a minimum or be resented otherwise. Since patients present the physician so constrained with problems that the physician regards as non-clinical and hence inappropriate, we have the setting for an unfortunate physician-patient encounter, leading to both an unhappy physician and an equally frustrated patient.

Psychiatry can sometimes be helpful here. It is the branch of medicine that specifically is interested in the problems that patients present to physicians that nonpsychiatric physicians often find frustrating and offputting: problems of communication, strong emotions, idiosyncratic ideas and beliefs, unreasonable expectations, noncompliant behavior, and so on. I have often said to psychiatry residents that "psychiatrists are physicians who see patients other physicians don't want to see," which is a facetious way to make the point.

All physicians can benefit from learning about the things that interest psychiatrists, and that is why every medical school curriculum requires a certain amount of experience with psychiatric patients. Certainly all psychiatry clerkships strive to help medical students become familiar with psychiatric thinking and the major psychiatric disorders, even though only a small percentage will ultimately specialize in psychiatry. In this, the psychiatric clerkship experience is like all other clinical rotations, which are designed to give medical students an introduction to a broad overview of clinical medicine. But not all such rotations place enough emphasis on the possibilities of incorporating into one's clinical out-look, to be used wherever one eventually will work, the central focus of psychiatry—an interest in and an approach to the patient's mental pro-cesses and behavior.

Like other medical practitioners, psychiatrists must be interested in the operations of different body systems in two parallel and sometimes highly correlated ways: the patient's subjective awareness and experi-ences and objective manifestations of organ function. Nearly all physi-cians recognize the essential importance of the patient's history for di-agnosis and treatment. The history is the patient's report of his or her experiences with health and illness, including the longitudinal course of symptoms and signs. It is embedded in a description of the individ-ual's family and social context, and related to the history of health and illness in other family members. It is not very often that the physician can perform optimally in the care of patients without such a history. In fact, typically, observations of the patient's physiology can only be prop-erly interpreted against the backdrop of the patient's history.

It is vital that the physician try to understand the patient's subjective experiences, including emotions, thoughts, perceptions, and beliefs about the illness and its treatment. This is especially true when the patient's illness is chronic or recurrent, or when it is associated with significant pain or disability, or if it appears to be life-threatening. It is what good clinical practice requires and what good clinical psychiatry depends upon. The clinical picture, the response to treatment, compliance, and many other matters of medical importance are influenced by the patient's mental and emotional state. This point is extremely important because it delin-eates the proper scope of clinical medicine and clinical psychiatry es-pecially. I have been arguing strongly that the medical model articu-lated here places an indispensable emphasis on the patient's inner experiences.

Psychiatric Education and Satisfactions in Medical Practice

Psychiatry is the branch of medicine that opens up the widest possibili-ties for very special and clinically appropriate close and trusting relation-ships with patients and sometimes even with their families. Psychiatrists can hope to see the confidence and trust of their patients develop, so that no experience and no concern, no matter how intimate and difficult, need be taboo. This is critically important in psychiatry, but it should be of great importance to all who enter one of the helping professions. Without such confidence and trust, our effectiveness will be lessened and our satisfactions reduced.

One aspect of practice that can be very satisfying is the cultivation of attitudes and skills designed to help patients learn how to recognize and talk about their experiences, including their thoughts, feelings, worries, fears, disappointments, anger and resentment, and so on. Interviewing patients offers never-ending challenges to one's ability to observe and, where appropriate, attempt to modify their communication, and even thinking, patterns. Many patients and relatives have difficulties presenting a coherent story about their illnesses, past and present. They may not be able to articulate clearly just what their complaints consist of, nor are they able to describe clearly the course or variation over time of their symptoms. Rather than become frustrated, or even angry, about such failures, psychiatrists must try to overcome them. Such communication difficulties are best viewed as clinically relevant, rather than as extraneous factors interfering with clinical practice.

Since psychiatrists, almost by definition, are interested in the ways patients communicate, think, perceive and relate to their worlds, and interpret what others say and do, they are likely to find talking to patients interesting and challenging. Psychiatrists are also very likely to be interested in the way patients feel about many things, experience emotions, approach their close relationships, and handle conflicts and frustrations, again making patients stimulating to work with. Finally, psychiatrists are interested in patients' temperament and personality, value systems, sexuality, and response sets and expectations. If the education and training of other physicians are suitably designed, they too should find something interesting in all patients.

The key to achieving this perspective is to be found in the approach to patients. Whether the principal problem is diagnostic or therapeutic, whether the patient is inarticulate or verbally skillful, whether the presenting picture involves disturbances in affect and mood (depression, anxiety, mania) or in thinking and belief (delusions, hallucinations) or impaired cognition (memory impairment, disorientation, confusion) or whether the patient is cooperative and wanting help or is resisting the whole idea of psychiatric difficulty, patients can be interesting for so many reasons that it is truly saddening when a physician fails to find them so. The only reasonable explanation is that the physician's initial interests and temperament were inappropriate for medicine or that the physician's preparation and training failed. The physician's initial attitude, education, and training, together with later reinforcements in practice, fostered so constricted and narrow a perspective about illness and medicine that the physician ends up not recognizing as properly clinical—and thus the physician's responsibility and challenge—many of the most interesting features of medical practice. Physicians who are able to do this are fortunate. They will have established one of the basic elements of an interesting and intellectually stimulating approach to all patients, regardless of specialty. Psychiatry can help students and residents not planning a career in psychiatry develop the attitudes and skills to accomplish this broader, more stimulating approach to clinical medicine.

The Role of Research in Medical Education

Psychiatry thus has a twofold responsibility in its educational and training programs: to teach the substance of clinical psychiatry, and to play a central role in making human thought, emotion, and behavior—in all of their richness—intellectually exciting for all physicians. The best way to work toward these goals is to make explicit to our students and trainees what we are hoping to accomplish, what our goals for them consist of. We must then approach all learning exercises with these goals in mind. We should also encourage all trainees to participate in some research—there is no truly satisfactory substitute for such experiences. Clinical research has a very special place in the education and training of individuals who are intending to concentrate on clinical medicine. Many fewer such individuals are likely to become involved in basic research because usually the focus in basic research seems more remote from questions of clinical interest than is true of clinical research. This should not be interpreted to mean that basic research is less important or not vitally relevant to our ultimate understanding about illness and health. It is simply a recognition of what is likely to be of *immediate* interest to those planning a clinical career.

Participation in a clinical research effort gives the medical student or resident an opportunity to understand the details of investigation that are impossible to grasp as well in any other way. All physicians must understand as much as possible about the basis of clinical practice. This means that each physician must distinguish between clinical practice based upon traditional clinical teaching and clinical practice based upon the findings from systematic and controlled studies. The idea is not to make full-time researchers out of all medical students and residents. Rather, it is to strengthen their clinical knowledge by increasing their sophistication concerning such knowledge, thus improving their functioning as clinicians.

Making such learning experiences available to students and residents requires a faculty that includes some individuals whose interests and experiences in clinical research permit them to serve as mentors. This has a number of very important implications. First, it implies that all psychiatry departments involved in education and training should be involved in research, at least to some extent.

Research and the Future of Psychiatry

This brings us to the very important question as to the appropriate place of research in psychiatry. Until recently, perhaps the last fifteen years, psychiatry placed a low priority on research. Only a few departments of psychiatry reflected a serious commitment to psychiatric research, at least as measured by the number of their researchers, the amount of space assigned to research activities, and the amount of money spent on research. In addition, there was very little encouragement of psychiatry residents to participate in ongoing investigation or to seriously consider a research career.

Over the past fifteen years or so, the situation has greatly improved. But it is still unsatifactory. A reasonably generous estimate is that only about twenty percent of all medical school departments of psychiatry have a strong commitment to research. We are talking about a few hundred individuals in psychiatry departments who are spending at least half their time in research of all kinds. If we assume that about two-thirds of these individuals are psychiatrists (in contrast to other disciplines) and add the research psychiatrists at the National Institute of

Mental Health, the National Institute of Alcohol Abuse and Alcoholism, and the National Institute of Drug Abuse, there may be no more than several hundred research psychiatrists in the United States.

By no criterion can this be regarded as a satisfactory level of commitment to research in a field as important as psychiatry. The frequency of disabling psychiatric disorders, their tendency to recurrence and chronicity, the associated family and social disruption, as well as the very high financial costs related to treatment and lost productivity, warrant a much greater effort.

Even though the number of dollars spent on research for each case of serious psychiatric disorder is only a tiny fraction of what is spent for each case of heart disease or each case of cancer, it is not very likely that parity will be achieved very soon. Estimates concerning research expenditures per patient are problematic at best, and perhaps dollars spent per case may not be a very good measure for determining how much should be spent. But it is one available measure and it indicates a very large gap. I would propose that psychiatric research should receive larger increases in new funding until the gap is less overwhelming.

What to do in the meantime? Psychiatry departments need a plan for developing research programs that will provide the intellectual base for entering upon a learned profession. The easiest way to begin is to initiate systematic clinical studies based upon the clinical work in the department. There is still a tremendous need for sophisticated studies concerning diagnosis, prognosis, treatment, and outcome. Most reported studies involve relatively small samples, thus precluding the answer to many significant questions. There is still much room to improve our methods for evaluating patients: eliciting their histories, describing their mental status examinations, increasing compliance with treatment, learning more about their day-to-day functioning, and so on.

Instituting systematic databases incorporating clinical information, developing effective understanding about statistical procedures and thinking, and establishing the positive attitudes toward such work are all within the capability of nearly every department. If the departmental leaders accept the essential role of an atmosphere encouraging investigation in the development of a modern educational and training program, they will be able to figure out ways to get started.

Once such a foundation has been laid, further developments can be added as additional resources become available. Epidemiologic studies can be initiated, their scope matched to resources. These can easily be tied to clinical studies. In both forms of research, medical students and residents can be recruited to expand the pool of active participants. Clinical studies will inevitably lead to ideas about brain phsyiology and development, which can set the stage for initating laboratory studies, perhaps relying at first on overlapping interests in other departments, such as pharmacology or neurobiology, which can make available mentors and collaborators and sometimes even facilities.

The Future of Psychiatry as a Specialty

What will the future of psychiatry be like if the viewpoint argued for in this book fails to prevail? I believe it will disappear as a medical specialty and be replaced by other mental health professions. One powerful reason is that other mental health professionals can provide psychotherapeutic interventions at a cost well below that of psychiatrists. To the extent that psychiatric practice is defined primarily by the provision of pscyhotherapeutic services, psychiatrists will find themselves severely disadvantaged in a marketplace where cost containment is a major driving force.

There is a certain irony in this. Psychoanalysis exerted great influence on the professional thinking and practice of the other mental health professions as well as on psychiatry. In fact, for a generation, psychoanalysis was the predominant theory shaping the training and thinking of students in all these professions. It is therefore not surprising that graduates from nonpsychiatric training programs placed primary emphasis in their practices on various forms of psychotherapy, gradually competing more and more with psychiatrists, nearly always at lower cost.

Related to these developments and accelerating them, Employee Assistance Programs (EAPs) directed by psychologists or social workers have been established in many business corporations. These programs were conceived to help employees with psychological problems, including substance abuse. Cost was an important reason for placing other mental health professionals in charge instead of psychiatrists. This has led to the referral of employees with such problems to other social workers and psychologists rather than to psychiatrists, primarily for psychotherapeutic treatment. Whether this has been the optimal treatment for many of these employees is certainly a question, but, thus far, any such doubts have had only limited impact.

Closely intertwined with these issues of professional competition is the fact that some people needing help for psychological problems feel less threatened by being referred to a psychologist or a social worker than to a psychiatrist. They fear that referral to a psychiatrist implies a "mental" problem, with the stigma that still clings to such conditions, while referral to one of the other mental health professionals implies a "problem in living" or in "stress management." These euphemisms that professionals bandy about represent more than an understandable desire to put the best face on any problem: they often reflect a limited understanding of the nature of psychiatric conditions.

Another recent political and legal development is the effort by psychologists to gain the legal right to admit patients to the hospital under their sole professional responsibility, so that they need not defer to any physician in the care of their patients. Psychologists have also tried to gain the legal right to prescribe psychoactive medications without the supervision of physicians. While some psychologists see little merit in the medical model and claim to be fully capable of handling all psychiatric conditions without need for medical experience, others argue that, without such medical experience and training, they should be permitted to do nearly everything that psychiatrists do, including prescribing medication and hospitalizing patients without medical supervision.

The medical model applied to psychiatric disorders carries with it many important social, economic, and political implications. To the extent that the model is persuasive as the best way to conceptualize and approach psychiatric problems, medical education and training are essential prerequisites for psychiatric practice. Under such circumstances, it makes little sense to give other mental health professionals functions that have traditionally been associated exclusively with the medical profession. While it is true that many individuals can be trained to perform specific and limited services that are considered medical, such as those carried out by physician assistants and nurse practitioners, there has been limited movement thus far in the direction of allowing such individuals to practice independently, free from all physician supervision. If patients need medical care, they should be the responsibility of duly trained physicians. If patients do not need medical intervention, or if they are not likely to benefit from such intervention, why should nonphysicians be allowed to carry out what are essentially medical procedures?

The central issues involve the nature of psychiatric disorders. Does optimal knowledge depend upon evolving biomedical science? A "no" answer is not really credible in view of what has been learned in the last twenty years about neurobiology and genetics. If the answer is "yes," does it make sense to have psychiatric patients treated by *independent* professionals who have not had medical education and training? Why should psychiatric patients be so handled when we would not agree to have cancer patients or heart patients or neurologic patients treated this way?

The future of psychiatry will be shaped by many forces, including economic, political, and scientific ones. I very much hope that scientific advances will prove to be the most influential. Growing knowledge of the brain's functions in carrying out mental processes and behavioral tasks, within an adaptive genotype-environment interaction that allows for individual variation, will make the difference in the long run. This implies that psychiatric education and training will be increasingly shaped by the medical model. It is another version of my argument for psychiatric research (Guze 1977).

The future of psychiatry depends greatly upon its leaders, especially its academic leaders. Their beliefs and commitments will, to a considerable extent, determine the future of the specialty. Leadership requires a vision and a program. These must be derived from a valid grasp of the field and its possibilities that will shape the education and training of medical students (most of whom will not become psychiatrists) and of psychiatric residents. If the medical model is not the basis for psychiatry's future, there appears to be little justification for a medical specialty concerned primarily with abnormal psychological manifestations.

8

Summing Up

The purpose of this book has not been to set forth our specialized and technical knowledge of psychiatric disorders, not to describe the diagnosis, treatment, etiology, pathogenesis, and epidemiology of each disorder. Instead, my aim has been to articulate as clearly and effectively as possible a strategy for thinking about psychiatric disorders. The model I have presented for conceptualizing an approach to these conditions is justified by its coherence and breadth. This model provides a legitimate place for all the currently recognized scientific concerns that are relevant to the understanding of psychiatric disorders. In addition, from the model's perspective, the presentation has included discussions about psychiatric education, training, and research; some of the frequently encountered pitfalls in psychiatric thinking; and with certain philosophical issues that psychiatry must consider.

My arguments can be subsumed under two main axioms. The first is that psychiatry makes more sense and will make the greatest progress by following the paths trod so successfully by the rest of medicine. This belief is encapsulated in the notion of the "medical model," which has been defined as using in psychiatry the intellectual traditions, basic concepts, and clinical as well as research strategies that have evolved in general medicine. These include systematic clinical description, systematic methods of examination, and the essential ideas of diagnosis, epidemiology, etiology, pathogenesis, response to interventions, natural history, and prognosis. The underlying assumption here, in general medicine as well as psychiatry, is that illnesses comprise a large number of different entities, which must be recognized, categorized, compared, and studied in systematic efforts to learn about their causes, the mechanisms of their various manifestations, their course and outcome, and their responses to different interventions.

The second axiom is that the brain is the organ of the mind, and that the future of psychiatry will depend increasingly upon growing understanding of the operations of the brain in carrying out those processes that are called higher brain functions, such as perceiving, thinking, learning, remembering, imagining—in other words, mental functions. Here too, the emphasis is on following the pathways of general medicine, where it has long been understood that medicine depends upon increasing knowledge of the body's anatomy and physiology. However, this emphasis on neurobiology as a central concern of psychiatry is imbedded in a very broad view of biology. It includes a fundamental belief that the study of all forms of life must include the essential perspective of *adaptation* as the touchstone for understanding. It builds upon evolution with its emphasis on the adaptation of species and includes the assumption that health and disease are different phases of the individual's adaptation to its complex environment: physical, cultural, familial, and interpersonal.

Furthermore, and very important, this approach to biology includes the recognition that the individual's inner life—hopes, fears, wishes, needs, fantasies, and feelings—is a vital part of the whole and needs to be studied clinically and physiologically. Because biology so conceived is very broad, one might say that psychiatry cannot be anything but biological. According to this view, one's feelings and thoughts are as biological as one's blood pressure or gastric secretion: feelings and thoughts are manifestations of the brain's operations just as blood pressure reflects the operations of the cardiovascular system and gastric secretion the stomach's function.

Psychiatry, as well as the rest of medicine, must be interested in such manifestations of the operations of different organs and body systems along two sometimes highly correlated paths: the patient's subjective experiences and the patient's objective physiology. Physicians have long recognized the great importance of the patient's complaints and history for diagnosis and treatment. The patient's history refers to the patient's report, supplemented by the reports of others, of the patient's experiences with health and illness, including the longitudinal course of symptoms and signs, imbedded in a description of the individual's familial and social context, and related to the history of health and illness in other family members. Physicans cannot perform optimally in caring for patients without such history. Indeed, very often, observations of the patient's physiology can only be properly interpreted in terms of the patient's history.

The model of thinking advocated here permits appropriately moti-vated and trained psychiatrists to pursue their special interests without disengaing from psychiatry's medical roots and without becoming de-railed from modern biomedical science. Clinical medicine, and espe-cially clinical psychiatry, cannot legitimately escape from a strong con-cern with the patient's subjective experience of illness, nor from a parallel concern with the interaction between the patient's illness and reaction to the illness and the patient's temperament and personality. Psychia-trists, by and large, understand this; other physicians are slowly coming to this understanding too. Clinical thinking must deal with these central matters, from both a practical and theoretical point of view. From a practical perspective, physicans need to be familiar with their patient's subjective experiences so as to deal with their medical problems more effectively. From a theoretical perspective, physicians who are not in-terested in their patients' sujective experiences will lack a full concep-tual grasp of medicine.

This entire book has been about strategic philosophical and scientific concepts. My thesis throughout has been that such concepts are fun-damentally important in shaping our approaches to psychiatric illnesses and psychiatric treatments. As we learn more about the etiology and pathogenesis of psychiatric conditions, confusion and controversy about these conceptual issues may diminish, but it is likely that some will continue to challenge us, since they are so intimately associated with religious and other cultural concerns about the nature of humankind and our place in the scheme of things. It does not seem likely, as some fear, that psychiatry will become "mindless."

To the contrary, the position proposed here rejects both a "mindless" and a "brainless" psychiatry. No modern biology can ignore the fact that mental processes—the mind—are the result of evolution, and thus must be studied and understood within a broad adaptive framework for explaining their nature, including their intimate, inseparable connec-tion with the brain. No modern psychiatry can ignore the substrate of the mind's operations: the brain. The model proposed here derives its main strengths and usefulness from the emphatic rejection of any need to choose between the mind and the brain when thinking about psychi-atric disorders.

At the same time, the many pitfalls encountered in thinking about psychiatric disorders have been emphasized. Not rarely, clinical obser-vations and even systematic studies fail to give proper attention to the need for appropriate controls to deal with investigator bias, the problems in achieving reliable and consistent measurements or descriptions, and the large number of potentially confounding variables that so often intrude into the study of humans.

Despite these hurdles, much has been learned about many psychiatric disorders that is valid and useful. Further, because knowledge in medicine, based upon proper studies, tends to be cumulative, there is reason to be optimistic about psychiatry's future. More sophisticated and better designed studies—in epidemiology, clinical practice, genetics, and neurobiology—will lead to more effective interventions and may even engender effective prevention strategies.

The medical model described here does not depend upon any specific etiological hypothesis. It can encompass social experiences as well as specific genes as etiological agents. It is based on the belief that psychiatry will progress most successfully by following the experiences of general medicine, upon which the model is explicitly patterned. A guide for teaching, practice, and research, it does not pretend to provide ready answers to the large number of questions we face every day. These answers will follow from careful research guided by the model.

Recognizing the importance of neurobiology is not equivalent to asserting that we know much about the etiology of most psychiatric disorders. Rather, it reflects the assumption that the more we learn about the way the brain works in supporting mental processes, the more we will understand about psychopathology.

Some psychiatrists, having considered the model presented here, argue that there is greater merit in using several models simultaneously: the psychodynamic, the sociological, and the biological, sometimes lumped together as the biopsychosocial model. All models, including the one I prefer, are devices for helping us think; as such, they can be a matter of taste. It is important, however, to differentiate the names of our models from the assumptions that underlie them and from the quality of the evidence in favor of the assumptions. The medical model incorporates the social environment as well as emotional states; it could be said, therefore, that the medical model described here is also biopsychosocial. I see advantages, however, in using the label "medical model" because it represents a comprehensive, integrated framework while emphasizing its derivation from general medical experience. Furthermore, its close integration with neurobiology emphasizes that understanding the brain is at the hub of our intellectual system.

One's conceptual approaches to psychiatric disorders are associated with major practical implications. This is an important point that warrants repetition. Many of these implications were discussed in the chapter on psychiatric education, training, and research. A different kind of ramification is to be seen in the way our health insurance system has dealt with coverage for psychiatric disorders: widespread retreat from previous efforts to treat psychiatric problems as all other medical problems are treated.

Today, only a rare insurance plan provides comparable coverage for psychiatric illnesses as for general medical illnesses. Higher deductibles, higher copayments, and fewer days of hospitalization or outpatient visits are the rule for psychiatric patients. The pattern is very difficult to rationalize, except for the explanation that insurance plans are trying to reduce their costs and keep premiums as low as possible. Most plans assume the public will tolerate discrimination in coverage against psychiatric illness because they believe that psychiatric disorders are not "real illnesses" and that they will always happen to other people. The unwary subscriber, usually with limited if any experience of psychiatric illness, is shocked and anguished when someone in the family develops severe depression or mania or schizophrenia and discovers that the copayment, for example, represents half of the total cost of the hospitalization, the current policy of many health insurance plans.

The point to emphasize here is that the explicit discrimination against mental illnesses, which can't be justified by the medical model, reflects the assumption or belief that mental illnesses are not true illnesses. If they are recognized as illnesses like all other medical conditions, a policy of discrimination against them makes no sense. Clearly the way one thinks about psychiatric disorders is not only of academic concern; directly and indirectly, it shapes industry and government policy about health insurance, sometimes with great impact on psychiatric patients and their families. We may have to control the growing costs of health care, but we should not do it by discriminating against a particular category of illness that can be as painful, disabling, and life-threatening as most other serious medical conditions, and that is often long-lasting and broadly pervasive in its manifestations.

I believe that the main reason for singling out psychiatric disorders for disproportionate cost savings is that most people still do not understand the reality, the extent, and the burdens of psychiatric conditions. Clinically signfiicant psychiatric disorders are very common, and this may be part of the problem. As insurance plans began to provide coverage for such illnesses, they were surprised and even overwhelmed by the large number of claims. They had not recognized how frequently such illnesses occur. Now that they have begun to appreciate the facts about this, they are trying to take advantage of the general public's relative ignorance to cut costs, at the expense of a very large number of people.

It makes no sense to discriminate against patients whose delusions and hallucinations are the result of the brain disorder called schizophrenia or whose intense excitement and severely impaired judgment are the result of the brain disorder called mania, while providing, as insurance companies do, for patients with similar clinical manifestations resulting from brain disorders called encephalitis or brain disorders based upon various endocrine abnormalities. Schizophrenia or mania or obsessive-compulsive disorder, to name only three examples, can be as disabling or destructive as any illness for which full insurance coverage is available. What rational basis for such discrimination can there be? Unless one falls back on a deliberate and arbitrary decision to exlude psychiatric disorders purely and simply to control costs without any consideration for the needs of the people covered by the insurance plan, one must conclude that the insurance companies do not consider psychiatric disorders to be valid medical conditions.

Psychiatric illnesses are real. They are associated with great suffering, disability, and premature death. Their victims and the families of victims deserve our genuine sympathy, compassion, and fairness.

References

Andreoli TE, Carpenter CCJ, Plum F, Smith LH Jr (editors). *Cecil's Essentials of Medicine*, WB Saunders, Philadelphia, 1986.

Boyd JH, Pulver AE, Stewart W. Season of birth: schizophrenia and bipolar disorder. Schizophrenia Bulletin 12:173–186, 1986.

Brady JV. Psychiatry and its poor relations: "Less than warmly embraced, more than misunderstood." J Nerv Ment Dis 176:581–584, 1988.

Brown GW, Harris T. *Social Origins of Depression*, Tavistock Publications, London, 1978.

Champion L. The relationship between social vulnerability and the occurrence of severely threatening life events. Psychol Med 20:157–161, 1990.

Changeaux J-P. *Neuronal Man. The Biology of Mind*, Pantheon Books, New York, 1985.

Charlton BG. A Critique of Biological Psychiatry. Psychol Med 20:3–6, 1990.

Churchland PS. *Neurophilosophy. Toward a Unified Science of the Mind/Brain*, MIT Press, Cambridge, Massachusetts, 1986.

Churchland PM, Churchland PS. Intertheoretic Reduction: A Neuroscientist's Field Guide. Seminars in the Neurosciences 2:249–256, 1990.

Cloninger CR. A unified biosocial theory of personality and its role in the development of anxiety states. Psychiatric Developments 3:167–226, 1986.

Cloninger CR. A systematic method for clinical description and classification of personality variance. A proposal. Arch Gen Psychiat 44:573–588, 1987.

Cloninger CR, Martin RL, Clayton P, Guze SB. A blind follow-up and family study of anxiety neurosis: Preliminary analysis of the St. Louis 500. In *Anxiety: New Research and Changing Concepts*, edited by DF Klein, J Rabkin, Raven Press, New York, 1981.

Crow TJ, Bal J, Bloom SR, Brown R, Bruton CJ, Colter N, Frith CD, Johnstone EC, Owens DGC, Roberts GW. Schizophrenia as an Anomaly of Development of Cerebral Asymmetry: A Post-Mortem Study and Proposal Concerning the Genetic Basis of the Disease. Arch Gen Psychiat 46:1145–1150, 1989.

Dalen P. *Season of Birth: A Study of Schizophrenia and Other Mental Disorders*, University of Göteborg, Göteborg, Sweden, 1975.

Damasio H, Damasio AR. *Lesion Analysis in Neuropsychology*, Oxford University Press, 1989.

Dawson DF. Letter to the Editor. Am J Psychiatry 135:1434–1435, 1978.

Dennett DC. *Elbow Room. The Varieties of Free Will Worth Wanting*, MIT Press, Cambridge, Massachusetts, 1984.

Dryja TP, Mukai S, Petersen R, Rapaport JM, Walton D, Yandell DW. Parental Origin of Mutations of the Retinoblastoma Gene. Nature 339:556–558, 1989.

Dunham HW. *Community and Schizophrenia*, Wayne State University Press, Detroit, 1965.

Early TS. The Left Striato-Pallidal Hyperactive Model of Schizophrenia. Proceedings of the VIII World Congress of Psychiatry. In *Psychiatry. A World Perspective, Volume 2*, Stefanis CN, Soldatos CR, Rabavilas AD (eds), Excerpta Medica, Amsterdam-New York-Oxford, 1990. (a)

Early TS. Left Globus Pallidus Hyperactivity in Right Sided Hemineglect in Schizophrenia. In *Schizophrenia: Origins, Processes, Treatment, and Outcome*, Cromwell RL (ed), Oxford University Press, New York, 1991. (b)

Eccles JC. *The Human Psyche*, Springer, Berlin, 1980.

Eccles JC. *Evolution of the Brain: Creation of the Self*, Routledge, London, 1989.

Edelman GM. *Neural Darwinism. The Theory of Neuronal Group Selection*, Basic Books, New York, 1987.

Edelman GM, Mountcastle VB. *The Mindful Brain: Cortical Organization and the Group-Selection Theory of Higher Brain Function*, MIT Press, Cambridge, Massachusetts, 1978.

Edelson M. *Psychoanalysis. A Theory in Crisis*, University of Chicago Press, Chicago, 1988.

Feighner JP, Robins E, Guze SB, Woodruff RA, Winokur G, Munoz R. Diagnostic criteria for use in psychiatric research. Arch Gen Psychiatry 26:57–63, 1972.

Feinstein AR. *Clinical Judgement*, Williams & Wilkins, Baltimore, 1967.

Feinstein AR. *Clinical Epidemiology*, WB Saunders, Philadelphia, 1985.

Feinstein AR, Pritchett J, Schimpff CR, Spitz H. The epidemiology of cancer therapy. I. Clinical problems of statistical surveys. Arch Internal Med 123:171–186, 1969. (a)

Feinstein AR, Pritchett J, Schimpff CR, Spitz H. The epidemiology of cancer therapy. II. The clinical course: Data, decision, and temporal demarcation. Arch Internal Med 123:323–344, 1969. (b)

Feinstein AR, Pritchett J, Schimpff CR, Spitz H. The epidemiology of cancer therapy. III. The management of imperfect data. Arch Internal Med 123:448–461, 1969. (c)

Feinstein AR, Pritchett J, Schimpff CR, Spitz H. The epidemiology of cancer therapy. IV. The extraction of data from medical records. Arch Internal Med 123:571–590, 1969. (d)

Frances A. Lecture presented at the annual meeting of the American Psychiatric Association, New York, May 1990.

Gabbard GO. The relevance of dynamic psychiatry in the 1990's. Psychiatric Times, April 1990. (a)

Gabbard GO. *Psychodynamic Psychiatry in Clinical Practice*, American Psychiatric Press, Washington, DC, 1990. (b)

Gazzaniga MS. *The Social Brain*, Basic Books, New York, 1985.

Geschwind N, Galaburda AM. *Cerebrolateralization*, MIT Press, Cambridge, Massachusetts, 1987.

Goldberg EM, Morrison SL. Schizophrenia and social class. Br J Psychiatry 109:785–802, 1963.

Goodman A. Organic Unity Theory: The Mind-Body Problem Revisited. Am J Psychiatry 148:553–563, 1991.

Goodwin DW, Guze, SB. *Psychiatric Diagnosis*, 4th Edition, Oxford University Press, New York, 1989.

Gottesman II, Shields J. *Schizophrenia. The Epigenetic Puzzle*, Cambridge University Press, Cambridge, 1982.

Gould SJ. *Wonderful Life. The Burgess Shale and the Nature of History*, WW Norton and Co, New York, 1989.

Grünbaum A. *The Foundations of Psychoanalysis,*. University of California Press, Berkeley, 1984.

Gruzelier J, Flor-Henry PP (editors). *Hemisphere Asymmetries of Function in Psychopathology*, Elsevier, Amsterdam, 1979.

Guze SB. The need for toughmindedness in psychiatric thinking. South Med J 63:662–671, 1970. (a)

Guze SB. The role of followup studies: Their contribution to diagnostic classification as applied to hysteria. Semin Psychiatry 2:392–402, 1970. (b)

Guze SB. The future of psychiatry: Medicine or social science? J Nerv Ment Dis 165:225–230, 1977.

Guze SB. The nature of psychiatric illness: Why psychiatry is a branch of medicine. Comprehensive Psychiat 19:295–307, 1978. (a)

Guze SB. Validating criteria for Psychiatric Diagnosis: The Washington University approach. In Akiskal HS, Webb WL (editors), *Psychiatric Diagnosis*, New York, SP Scientific and Medical Books, 1978. (b)

Guze SB. Can the practice of medicine be fun for a lifetime? JAMA 241:2021–2023, 1979.

Guze SB. Psychosomatic medicine: A critique. Psychiatric Developments 2:23–30, 1984.

Guze SB. Psychotherapy and the etiology of psychiatric disorders. Psychiatric Developments 3:183–193, 1988.

Guze SB. Biological psychiatry: Is there any other kind? Psychological Medicine 19:315–323, 1989. (a)

Guze SB. Diagnosis in psychiatry: Philosophical and conceptual issues. Presented at Symposium on Clinical Research in Depression and Schizophrenia at the University of Pittsburgh, April 21–22, 1989. (b) To be published in the Proceedings.

Guze SB. Secondary depression: observations in alcoholism, Briquet's syndrome, anxiety disorder, schizophrenia, and antisocial personality. A form of comorbidity? In *The Psychiatric Clinics of North America*, volume 13 RB Wesner and G Winokur (editors), WB Saunders Company, 1990, pages 651–659.

Guze SB, Cloninger CR, Martin RL, Clayton PJ. A follow-up and family study of schizophrenia. Arch Gen Psychiat 40:1273–1276, 1983.

Guze SB, Cloninger CR, Martin R, Clayton PJ. Alcoholism as a medical disorder. Comprehensive Psychiatry 27:501–510, 1986.

Guze SB, Helzer JE. The medical model and psychiatric disorders. In Cavenar JO, Editor, *Psychiatry*, Philadelphia, JB Lippincott Company, 1985, Chapter 51, pages 1–8.

Guze SB, Murphy GE. An empirical approach to psychotherapy: The agnostic position. Am J Psychiatry 120:53–57, 1963.

Guze SB, Woodruff RA, Clayton PJ. Secondary affective disorders: A study of 95 cases. Psychol Med 1:426–428, 1971.

Hundert EM. *Philosophy, Psychiatry and Neuroscience*, Oxford University Press, New York, 1989.

Kandel ER, Schwartz JH. *Principles of Neural Science*, 2nd Edition, Elsevier, New York, 1985.

Karasu TB. Psychotherapies: an overview. Am J Psychiatry 134:851–863, 1977.

Karasu TB. The specificity versus non-specificity dilemma: toward identifying therapeutic change agents. Am J Psychiatry 143:687–695, 1986.

Karasu TB. New frontiers in psychotherapy. J Clin Psychiatry 50:46–49, 1989.

Karasu TB. Toward a clinical model of psychotherapy for depression, I: Systematic comparison of three psychotherapies. Am J Psychiatry 147:133–147, 1990.

Kendell RE. *The Role of Diagnosis in Psychiatry*, Blackwell, Oxford, 1975.

Lewis MS. Age incidence in schizophrenia; Part I. The season of birth controversy. Schizophrenia Bulletin 15:59–73, 1989. (a)

Lewis MS. Age incidence in schizophrenia: Part II. Beyond age incidence. Schizophrenia Bulletin 15:75–80, 1989. (b)

Lewis MS. *Res Ipsa Loquitor:* The Author Replies, Schizophrenia Bulletin 16:17–28, 1990.

Lewontin RC. Letter to the Editor. *The New York Review of Books*, May 31, 1990.

Lifton RJ. *The Nazi Doctors*, Basic Books, New York, 1986.

Margolis H. *Patterns, Thinking, and Cognition*, University of Chicago Press, Chicago, 1988.

Maser JD, Cloninger CR (editors). *Comorbidity of Mood and Anxiety Disorders*, American Psychiatric Press, Washington, DC, 1990.

Mayr E. *The Growth of Biological Thought. Diversity, Evolution, and Inheritance*, Harvard University Press, Cambridge, Massachusetts, 1982.

Mayr E. *Toward a New Philosophy of Biology*, Harvard University Press, Cambridge, Massachusetts, 1988.

Meehl PE. Appraising and Amending Theories: The Strategy of Lakatosian Defense and Two Principles that Warrant It. Psychological Inquiry 1:108–141, 1990.

Mellon CD, Clark LD. A Developmental Plasticity Model for Phenotypic Variation in Major Psychiatric Disorders. Perspectives in Biology and Medicine 34:35–43, 1990.

Murphy G, Guze SB, King L. Urinary excretion of 5-hydroxyindoleacetic acid in chronic alcoholism. JAMA 182:565, 1962.

Myers JM. *Cures by Psychotherapy*, Praeger Publishers, New York, 1984.

Pardo JV, Pardo P, Raichle ME. Human brain activation during dysphoria. Soc for Nueroscience Abstracts 17:664, 1991.

Pearlson GD, Ross CA, Lohr WD, Rovner BW, Chase GA, Folstein MF. Association between family history of affective disorder and the depressive syndrome of Alzheimer's disease. Am J Psychiatry 147:452–456, 1990.

Penfield W, Roberts L. *Speech and Brain-Mechanisms*, Princeton University Press, Princeton, New Jersey, 1959.

Philpot M, Rottenstein M, Burns A, Geoffrey D. Season of birth in Alzheimer's disease. Br J Psychiatry 155:662–666, 1989.

Popper KR, Eccles JC. *The Self and Its Brain*, Springer-Verlag, London, 1977.

Posner MI (editor). *Foundations of Cognitive Science*, MIT Press, Cambridge, Massachusetts, 1989.

Posner MI, Petersen SE, Fox PT, Raichle ME. Localization of cognitive operations in the human brain. Science 240:1627–1631, 1988.

Pulver AE, Stewart W, Carpenter WT Jr, Childs B. Risk factors in schizophrenia: season of birth in Maryland USA. Br J Psychiatry 143:389–396, 1983.

Purves D, Lichtman JW. *Principles of Neural Development*, Sinauer Associates, Sunderland, Massachusetts, 1985.

Reiss D, Plomin R, Hetherington E. Genetics and Psychiatry: An Unheralded Window on the Environment. Am J Psychiatry 143:283–291, 1991.

Robins E. *The Final Months*, Oxford University Press, New York, 1981.

Robins E, Guze SB. Establishment of diagnostic validity in psychiatric illness: Its application to schizophrenia. Am J Psychiatry 126:983–987, 1970.

Robins E, Guze SB. Classification of affective disorders: The primary-secondary, the endogenous-reactive, and the neurotic-psychotic concepts. In Williams TA, Katz MM, Shield JA, Jr (editors), *Recent Advances in the Psychobiology of the Depressive Illnesses*. NIMH, DHEW Publication No 70-9053, 1972, pages 283–293.

Rosenberg A. *Philosophy of Social Science*, Westview Press, Boulder, 1988.

Rosenhan DL. On being sane in insane places. Science 179:250–258, 1973.

Ruse M. *Taking Darwin Seriously*, Basil Blackwell, Oxford, 1986.

Sawaguchi T, Goldman-Rakic PS. DI dopamine receptors in prefrontal cortex: involvement in working memory. Science 251:947–950, 1991.

Scadding JG. The semantic problems of psychiatry. Psychol Med 20:243–248, 1990.

Scriver CR. An evolutionary view of disease in man. Proceedings of the Royal Society of London (series B) 220:273–298, 1984.

Scriver CR, Beaudet AL, Sly WS, Valle D (editors). *The Metabolic Basis of Inherited Disease*, second edition, McGraw-Hill, New York, 1989.

Siegel GJ, Agranoff BW, Albers RW, Molinoff TB (editors). *Basic Neurochemistry*, Raven Press, New York, 1989.

Skinner BF. *Cumulative Record*, Appleton-Century-Crofts, New York, 1959.

Snyder SH. *Drugs and the Brain*, Scientific American Libraries, New York, 1986.

Sokal RR. Classification: purposes, principles, progress, prospects, Science 185:1115–1123, 1974.

Spence DP. *Narrative Truth and Historical Truth*, WW Norton and Co, New York, 1982.

Spence DP. *The Freudian Metaphor*, WW Norton and Co, New York, 1987.

Sulloway FJ. *Freud, Biologist of the Mind*, Basic Books, New York, 1979.

Szasz TS. *The Myth of Mental Illness*, Hoeber-Harper, New York, 1961.

Szasz TS. The ethics of suicide. Antioch Review 31, Spring 1971.

Szasz TS. Mental illness as a metaphor, Nature 242:305–307, 1973.

Szasz TS. The myth of psychotherapy. Am J Psychotherapy 28:517–526, 1974.

Szasz TS. Psychiatric justice. Br J Psychiatry 154:864–869, 1989.

Tennant C. Life events and psychological morbidity: the evidence from prospective studies. Psychol Med 13:483–486, 1983.

Tennant C. Parental loss in childhood. Arch Gen Psychiat 45:1045–1050, 1988.

Tennant C, Bebbington P. The social causation of depression: a critique of the work of Brown and his colleagues. Psychol Med 8:565–575, 1978.

Tennant C, Bebbington P, Hurry J. Parental death in childhood and risk of adult depressive disorders: a review. Psychol Med 10:289–299, 1980.

Whitehorn JC. Psychodynamic approach to the study of psychoses. In *Dynamic Psychiatry*, edited by F Alexander and H Ross, University of Chicago Press, Chicago, 1952.

Woodruff RA, Murphy GE, Herjanic M. The natural history of affective disorders. 1. Symptoms of 72 patients at the time of index hospital admissions. J Psychiat Res 5:255–263, 1967.

Wyngaarden JB, Smith LH Jr (editors). *Cecil's Textbook of Medicine, 18th Edition*, WB Saunders, Philadelphia, 1988.

Young JZ. *Programs of the Brain*, Oxford University Press, Oxford, 1978.

Young JZ. *Philosophy and the Brain*, Oxford University Press, Oxford, 1987.

Index